Wendy

My Brother's Keeper:
A Caregiver's Story

Wendy Mac Ewan Kroger

BLACK ROSE
writing™

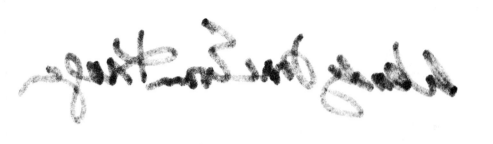

ISBN: 978-1-61296-771-4
PUBLISHED BY BLACK ROSE WRITING
www.blackrosewriting.com

Printed in the United States of America
Suggested retail price $16.95

My Brother's Keeper: A Caregiver's Story is printed in Minion Pro
Cover Painting by Tracy MacEwan, 'Exit, Stage Right"
36"x36" oil and wax on canvas
https://www.tracymacewan.com

First to my brother, Tracy, who is the most courageous and stubborn person I have ever met.

My heart is full of thanks to the people who gave so much to help Tracy – and me:

My daughter, Alison,

All my superlative supportive friends in Beaverton and Lincoln City,

The Amazing Professionals: Oregon Health Sciences University (OHSU) doctors, Neurosciences Intensive Care Unit and Kohler Pavilion Acute Care staff; Jackie in Finance; OHSU Physical Therapist, Andy; Rehabilitation Institute of Oregon (RIO) Therapists Val, Pete and Bernadette; and Speech Therapists, Daria (Legacy) and Katie (Forest Grove Rehabilitation Center); RN/massage therapist, Cheryl; Good Samaritan Clinic doctors Whitman and Smith; long-time friend, Dr. Allan Mandell.

And Bill.

My Brother's Keeper:
A Caregiver's Story

Table of Contents

Foreword

This is my story of the last five years. Many people are part of it. My hope is that people who become inadvertent caregivers to someone they love will benefit from what I learned along the way.

The reason for the excruciating detail in parts of this story about my brother's stroke is that nothing much goes as planned -- especially if you are the one doing the planning and you don't know much about what you are doing. Often I fell several steps back before I could take a step forward. You'll understand what I mean about "excruciating detail" when you get to the sections about speech, student loans, and the Internal Revenue Service. I want to share what I learned. I discovered that, with a few exceptions, I could find the assistance I needed. Mostly, people want to help. I just needed to ask the *right* questions of the *right* people in the *right* place. And never to give up.

Without my brother, this would not be *my* story. I haven't written his story. I wouldn't dare to try.

There are stellar professionals out there. There are some not so much. My job as a caregiver was to find the stellar ones and get around the others. Luckily I found some great ones early -- they proved to me that great ones exist. Keeping my place in a line until I had either an answer or a specific suggestion of exactly where to go next helped move everything along. I became fearless about telephoning anyone I thought might help -- including the Governor's office and my congressional representative.

If you are reading this, please, please get a medical and financial Power of Attorney for yourself. You don't need it if you're dead. It's critical to you if you are alive.

And, finally, whenever you come across people who identify themselves as "caregiver," please do something nice for them. I'm afraid most of them are quietly drowning. They are the unsung heroes of today's America.

Part 1:
What Just Happened?

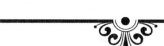

Chapter 1:
June 20, 2011:
The Day Everything Changed

June always has been my favorite month: celebrating birthdays and our anniversary, and this year we marked our granddaughter's high-school graduation. I love the gentle Pacific Northwest spring: mist holding such a splendid color of green. The garden is gorgeous; the air soft. In the Northwest, June is a month of promise for those of us who love the outdoors. And, for those who are gardeners, we already have been hard at work beginning in early spring primping and plumping, planting our special plants and seeds that still have perfection within them: everything is still possible. Gardeners are the ultimate optimists.

After spending the afternoon playing bridge with friends, I sat at our kitchen table with Bill, my husband, and told him of all we had talked about and how we had laughed at the silliest things. Bill was still unable to get out on his own, having torn his quadricep tendon from his kneecap in March. I tried to bring a little color into his life with my friends' stories since he spent much of each day at his computer and doing physical therapy and rehabilitation exercises. Bill was telling me that he'd been working and had heard back from Tracy, my brother, in mid-afternoon about the changes Bill wanted made on his website. Bill retired from the U.S. Army as a lieutenant colonel and is active in various veteran's organizations. The website for the local Military Officers Association of America (MOAA) chapter was Bill's baby. Bill had fought hard to move his local chapter into the modern communication age, and with Tracy's help and expertise, he'd gotten it to the point that it won a national award.

My cell phone rang. It was Kelly, a remarkable glass artist, sweet soul and very close friend of Tracy, who like my brother, lived on the Oregon Coast, a little more than one hundred miles away.

"Hi Kelly, what a surprise. Is everything okay?"

"Well, not really. It's Tracy. We are at the emergency room at Lincoln City Hospital and they are getting ready to put him on Life Flight to transfer him to OHSU Hospital in Portland." The enormity of what she just said did not register.

I asked, "Why would they be doing that?" I would more likely have believed a statement such as "He's just boarding the first passenger flight to Mars." Tracy is an artist and photographer, living precisely where he wants; he's in great shape: he exercises regularly, walks miles every day, eats healthy food, never smoked, drinks sparingly, is a careful driver.... I concluded that somehow, she had just got it all wrong.

I asked her, inanely since she is a great and close friend of my brother's, are you sure it's Tracy? She tried to explain but all I heard was, "He's sick... someone found him at the gym... he was outside... Silkie (who's that, I wondered?) wouldn't let him go home... they called an ambulance because he couldn't talk or walk... brain scan... now they say they think blood is leaking in his brain... maybe a stroke... his blood pressure is sky high... he needs more help than he can get here so they are Life Flighting him to their Trauma One Hospital in Portland..." She was trying to be very calm, but her tight voice was followed by a sob.

I looked at my phone. What was wrong with it? Bill looked at me very quizzically and asked, "What's happened?"

"It's Kelly," I said. "She says there's something wrong with Tracy and he's coming to Portland." Bill asked when he was arriving. I thought, "That's a good question..." In turn, I asked Kelly and she said, "I think it will take a couple of hours after they get all situated in the helicopter. They will land on the roof at OHSU." I asked if she was coming with him, realizing later how idiotic that was: there's so little room in a medical helicopter, they can barely fit in the patient. She said, "No." I told her we would be at OHSU to meet him. OHSU is Oregon Health Sciences University, the state's premier medical teaching university, which also is a first-rate Trauma One hospital serving many of Oregon's outlying smaller communities. After I hung up, I realized all the things I hadn't asked and all the things I should have said like, "Thank you." It must have been excruciating for her to make that phone call.

My mind was in a whirl. Thoughts cascaded all over themselves in no order whatever. Who should we notify? Of what? I didn't know anything yet.

What should we do? How, exactly do we get to OHSU and where should we park?

I stood up and turned from the table, but I didn't' know where I was going or what I was planning to do. I stopped and said, "We have to get to OHSU." Bill reached out and gently pulled me back into my chair. He said, "Tell me what's going on."

I repeated what Kelly had said, garbling it badly because I kept interjecting questions for which there were no answers. Questions like, "Why" and "How?" It's a good thing Bill had been a news reporter. It's the only way he must have made sense out of what I was saying. When he slowed me down with more down-to-Earth questions such as, "When do we need to be at OHSU?" I lashed out because he was slowing me down. I had to rush but I had no immediate direction. He said, "We'll be there. What do we need to do before we go?"

How do you get ready for something about which you know nothing? I felt as if the passage of time had fallen into a cold molasses bath. Everything had slowed down, and even sounds were odd, warped by being dialed down. We waited a very long two hours while Tracy traveled over the Coast Range from Lincoln City to Portland, a distance of about 120 miles. I started asking more questions, having no answers and trying to make sense out of the situation: We just saw him last week when we celebrated my birthday with him and friends at my favorite restaurant and he was fine. What could have happened? He's just 57 years old; how could he have had a stroke? That's what happens to old people. Will he be okay in the helicopter? What if they can't stabilize him? Is there a nurse on board? Or, a doctor? Should we call OHSU yet to see where we should meet the helicopter? Would we be at the hospital all night? Maybe I should get out extra cat food for our kitties, just in case. Bill had just gotten an email from Tracy this afternoon. I looked at it and could read nothing either sinister or prescient in it: no clues as to what was going to happen to him in less than two hours.

Finally, we could leave. It felt as if I'd been held back until now, and the gun starting the race had finally been fired. Bill had Googled OSHU, so we'd know where we were going. It helped but the substantial road construction made it more confusing. I drove because Bill couldn't. The temporary handicap parking sticker we had because of his knee was a blessing. We came in a back door that became our regular entry: I didn't find the "real" front entrance until many days later. We didn't wander long before we saw a staff person and I asked how to get to the roof to meet the helicopter that was coming in about 8:30 tonight. He smiled a very nice smile and said that usually the only people who went to the roof to meet Life Flight were medical staff. He asked a few more questions and suggested where to go to wait for information. After we checked in to the waiting room, we were told they would let us know when the helicopter arrived. Life Flight arrived about 8:45 p.m. and Tracy was taken immediately and directly for examination. We waited. Other families were in the waiting room that night. All of us were waiting to hear something, desperately hoping it would be something good. As the night progressed, I realized I hadn't eaten anything for dinner and I was hungry. We got directions to the cafeteria and I ate a big slice of pizza a little before midnight. Back in the waiting room, we checked in. There were signs in the waiting room discouraging falling asleep on the couches. But by midnight, people were doing just that.

A little before 2 a.m., a doctor came to talk to us. We didn't realize it at the time, but we had started down the road that many families and friends travel when loved ones suffer traumatic medical events. It was at this point that we began our serious medical education. The doctor said they had examined Tracy and were attempting to get his vital signs stabilized sufficiently so he could undergo brain surgery early in the morning. He had had a CT scan and an angiogram, among other tests, which indicated the presence, size and location of a blood clot and the potential location of a hemorrhage in the brain. The clot was so big, they were unable to determine the exact location of the leak without surgery. The tests also had indicated there was nothing wrong with his arterial or venal blood system in his brain – which was a good thing. We nodded our heads as if we understood what we had just been told. I thought maybe Bill really did know what all that meant. He thought the same about me. We reconnoitered later. Surgery was planned for 5:15 a.m. Its estimated duration was four-plus hours with additional time in recovery. The doctor encouraged us to go home and get some sleep. No one would be allowed to see Tracy. I asked if the doctor would tell him we were there. He smiled and said, "Sure."

We retraced our steps out the mystery door to the parking area. The car magically was still there. The night was cool and very dark away from the lights. It was quiet until an ambulance siren shredded the night. We drove back down what's called "Pill Hill" in Portland and found our way home. We went to bed but didn't sleep.

Chapter 2:
I Don't Know Anything and
I Need to Know Everything...

Early the next morning, trying to spring to life by drinking several cups of coffee, I let my mind roam. My thoughts were structured by my questions of the previous day: "how?" "why?" and "what happened?" The quizzically smiling face of my much younger brother danced in my head. I kept trying to find some clue, but none came for me to pounce upon, saying, "Aha! That's what happened."

We called immediate family and Kelly to let them know what little we knew. And then Bill and I returned to the same waiting room we had left a few hours before. This time, our daughter, Alison, was with us. As we drove back up "Pill Hill," it struck me: Doernbecher Children's Hospital is part of OHSU and one of the places where Sherry had been cared for so many years ago during her long and ultimately fatal battle with brain cancer. Sherry was my little sister who died when she was eight. I was ten. Tracy was born two years later. I hadn't been back to this area since Sherry died... until last night.

We timed our return to the hospital to when we thought Tracy would be out of surgery. He was in surgery for about four hours and would spend the remainder of the day coming back from the deep anesthesia and sedation needed for surgery. As we continued to wait, trying not to speculate on much of anything, a continuous procession of Tracy's friends from Lincoln City started to arrive. Much later that day, medical staff removed the breathing tube, which made his life much more comfortable. Tracy was moved to the Neurosciences Intensive Care Unit (ICU) where he would spend the next 16 days.

When I first saw Tracy in the Neurosciences ICU, I counted 17 tubes attached to his body. I had never been in such a place. It felt cold. It was very efficient; no frivolous extras. The only colors, I recall, were on a TV screen with someone talking on it and in a plastic tube draining blood and spinal fluid from my brother's head. Sound was mechanical: the hushed voices on the loudspeakers sounded metallic. Things gurgled, machines measuring vital signs pinged and bonged, pumps slurped, wet mops swished on the floor in the corridor outside the partially closed door to his room. A tall window bare of any adornment faced the side of another building and let in a little gray light. Irrationally, I wanted to change something, anything, to make this place warmer for Tracy. I asked that they change the TV channel from talking to one showing bright colored fish swimming across the screen.

Doctors and staff were in almost constant attendance. If they were not in the room working with Tracy, they were looking at the computer screen hooked up to his monitors. They circled his bed on their various missions, checking vital signs and asking him to perform many tasks. It seemed a hive of constant low-level activity. On the first day after surgery, he followed commands such as moving his toes when asked. He recognized us when we came next to his bed. He smiled when he saw us. When asked his name, he said "Tracy." He was unable to put together a sentence. He could not find words. He appeared unable to follow a thought from beginning to end. But he recognized us and smiled. I figured I could go a long way on that. In the days to come, staff would learn that each day there would be a complete circle of caring friends and family around Tracy. They would look in and see an entire ring of people around his bed. Very politely, but very firmly, they would ask us to take turns. Tracy's room became Noah's Ark: two loving people at a time.

I felt how I imagine a schizophrenic might feel: split. I was in the present but I saw Tracy in a tumbling kaleidoscope of bits and pieces of our lives. I saw him as a happy two-year-old sitting in the center of a big table in the school cafeteria while I and other freshmen Pep Club members made sandwiches around him for the football team. He was our mascot. He always came with me to Friday night Pep Club activities. I saw him in summertime when I took care of him each year for the summer when school was out. One summer, I crawled from the dormer window in my second-story bedroom across our steep roof into his dormer window because mom had sent him to bed while it was still light. I figured if it was light outside, who wanted to sleep? We made blanket tents and played for hours. Mom and Dad had Tracy after my sister died. Mom had a rough delivery, but she always told me that she had Tracy for *me*. He was mine. I believed her. Once when mom chastised Tracy for swearing (he was three) and I laughed, Dad said, "If someone drove up in a cab and said Tracy had just killed 36 people, Wendy would want to know what they did to make him mad." When he was eight-years-old, Tracy became desperately ill with spinal meningitis. He couldn't return to school for months, so he came to live with me to regain his strength and I got to fatten him up. My son was born during that time, and Tracy loved just watching the new baby. As the days ahead unfolded, they were colored by my memories. There was never a question of what I would do for Tracy. The single question was could I do *enough* for him so he could come back to us. I hope everyone has at least one person in their lives who they unreservedly love. While it can be heartbreaking, excruciating or terrifying, it is also the supreme joy of living.

When we saw the doctors during rounds, we asked about the surgery. Surgery had been successful: the large clot had been removed and the point of hemorrhage repaired. There was now a hole in the back of his head where the bone had been cut away to reach the clot. They were a little less happy, however, with the fact that most of the blood that had drained into the brain was still there. As they explained, brain tissue and blood are not supposed to touch each other. What I got from their explanation is that blood is acidic and the concern is that it eats away at blood vessels in the brain, hence the need to remove it as quickly as possible so there would be no repeat "incidents." They also had been hopeful that the ventricle which had been pressed down by the blood clot would "bounce back" quickly after surgery. It was not going as well as they had hoped because blood in the brain was continuing to put pressure on the ventricle. The tube they installed was to act as a siphon and an overflow valve. Of the several unknowns they talked about, one stood out for me: They were paying very close attention to Tracy's brain which had been thoroughly beaten up, and they would be watching for additional edema or swelling over the next four to five days. They said they just had no idea what might still happen. Bill and I were told that they were still trying to discern what was going on with his unstable blood pressure. We again did a lot of nodding our heads up and down. We had just heard many more new words – or in some cases, words we hadn't heard since high-school health class. We had decided earlier that if either of us didn't understand something, we were going to ask… and keep on asking until it made sense to us.

I sized up one of the doctors as looking more approachable than some of the others. I asked him several questions. He didn't disappoint. I started with, "What, exactly, is a stroke, and did my brother have one?" He said there are two basic types of strokes: the first, and less common, is hemorrhagic, which is a blow-out of one or more blood vessels or, as had occurred in Tracy's case, an intracerebral hemorrhage which occurs when a blood vessel bursts and bleeds into the tissue deep within the brain. The other, more common, stroke is an ischemic stroke, where blood clots come together in the blood stream, travel to various places in the body or brain, settle in and block the flow of blood, causing tissue to die from lack of nourishment. And, yes, my little brother had suffered an intracerebral hemorrhagic stroke in the cerebellum apparently brought on by undiagnosed chronic high blood pressure. I asked how to spell cerebellum because I had no real idea what or where it was. I had to refrain from laughing… something I'm pretty sure the doctor would not have appreciated. But I had a sudden flashback to a friend's mother who, when playing the game of Trivial Pursuit, answered the question, "Where is the medulla oblongata," with "Italy." I thought maybe the cerebellum was somewhere near the medulla oblongata, and with my lack of sleep, I thought it not impossible that they were both, indeed, in Italy. I've been told I should never play poker: I mirror what I'm thinking and am unable to keep a straight face. The doctor looked at me closely, made a note and said he was sending some information about strokes and blood pressure to Tracy's room. I should read it.

Medical jargon. I told myself to settle down and concentrate. After all, how complicated could it be? I'd had years of practice with bureaucratic jargon, having worked many years at various levels of government, managing and then evaluating jobs and training programs and writing investigative and audit reports in Washington, D.C. I'd overseen the production of several years' worth of semi-annual reports to Congress from the U.S. Labor Department's Inspector General. I'd taken many a deep dive into complicated minutia to ferret out what the findings actually were and gone on to interpret and write what I found for the benefit of the public. Surely, I could do the same for myself.

I was about to find out what an amazing bunch of friends Tracy has. Within twenty-four hours of his "event," one industrious 18-year-old named Harry had created a Facebook page called "Support for Tracy," which helped me immensely because I could write one post, instead of individual emails or make several telephone calls, and everyone -- friends nearby and relatives across the country -- could see it. Harry along with Jane, Robin and Kelly became the Administrators of this very active page.

Jane and Robin are from the Oregon coast and each in her own way seeks and reflects on the meaning of life. Jane reaches for it through a camera lens and Robin writes, acts and teaches. Both are long-time friends of Tracy's. Robin became the appointments director because so many people were coming and seeing Tracy. She had potential visitors sign up on his Facebook page, noting when they wanted to visit. She kept it to two people a visit. Some knew they would drive more than 100 miles and not see him for various reasons, but still they signed up and came. The Intensive Care Unit (ICU) waiting room became the greeting place: hugs, prayers, questions, updates. Tears and laughter were plentiful, because no one who knew Tracy could keep from smiling or laughing for long. Everyone brought something of themselves that they shared with Tracy as they held his hand or massaged his feet: pictures, music, funny stories. Jane and Kelly went to his house and packed two backpacks full of things they thought he might want: glasses, clothing, his iPod. They brought them to me and I started crying when I opened the first one. It smelled of Tracy.

We all learned that to get into the ICU area, one went through the process of picking up the wall phone outside, identifying oneself, asking to enter. Sometimes we were told "not now," or "in a few minutes," but we often were allowed to enter even though they were working on him. We also knew to squirt anti-bacterial hand sanitizer on our hands before we pushed the big gray button to activate the buzzer inside. Someone would then let us in, and we made our way around the nurses' station to his room. Sometimes the door was open; sometimes it was partly closed. There wasn't much extra space in his cubicle, so we tried very hard to make ourselves small and stay out of the way.

On the first evening Tracy was in the ICU, Tracy's nephew and my son, Mitch, along with his daughter Haylee and son Trenton, came to see him. Like all healthy people, who never see the inside of an ICU, they looked around, eyes wide, and retreated into quiet conversations among themselves. In this awkward moment, Bill said brightly, "Well, he looks pretty normal." Alison, our daughter, swung her head around and asked, "Normal? You think seventeen tubes in his body is normal?" After this icebreaker, Mitch and his kids re-engaged because they wanted some assurance that the Tracy lying there in that bed was really the irreverent, funny and warm Tracy they knew and loved and had just seen a few weeks ago. Trenton was dressed in his Reedville Little League baseball uniform, and the cleats on his shoes rang out on the floor when he walked. Mitch is a superlative baseball dad: he got his love of baseball from Tracy, passed it on to his son, and here was Trenton, in uniform in Tracy's room. Haylee, the recent high school graduate who plans to be a dentist, and her dad had a lively conversation aimed at Tracy. The gist was, "Hey, he doesn't look so bad. He's probably faking it." Tracy quietly said something. They leaned in and heard, "Scumbags."

The next morning, Tracy was unable to tell us his name. The nurse asked him again what his name was; he moved his head "No." He could not follow commands. He didn't wiggle his toes. He could say no words. He was apparently exhausted and physically more uncomfortable. But when I asked him if he remembered seeing Haylee the night before, he smiled and nodded his head, "Yes." I was getting "schooled" in the roller coaster of serious medical events: highs, lows, desperate fear, snatching and holding close any good news, denying that anything awful had happened, imbibing any information I could find. And realizing I had no control whatever.

Three days after his stroke, he had regressed: he was unable to talk or follow commands. Staff indicated it was likely because of the swelling caused by his brain being pummeled by the pooling blood. He also had developed pneumonia. He complained of back pain and seemed agitated and uncomfortable. The good news: he still recognized us, and the medical staff believed they were getting better control of his blood pressure. I noted the recurring theme of "uncontrolled high blood pressure." Knowing nothing about it, I asked the medical staff what symptoms he must have had that we should have looked for. They said it is often dubbed "The Silent Killer" precisely because there are no apparent symptoms. They wanted the blood pressure low so there's less chance of another blood vessel hemorrhaging. Tracy was sleeping most of the time. Partly that was his natural healing mechanism, but also it was partly because of medication. As one nurse said, "there's a real need for him to rest and no real need for him to remember his discomfort or fear when he leaves here. It would serve no purpose." Checking back later that night, I found that Tracy was still agitated, had a substantial amount of back pain, and his blood pressure was still elevated. Staff was trying various medications to bring down the blood pressure and alleviate his discomfort. At different times I asked what his blood pressure was. I don't recall ever hearing an exact set of numbers. To be truthful, I didn't understand what the different numbers meant anyway. I retained and made sense of words instead of numbers, so I heard them tell me that it was "very high," or, that his blood pressure was so unstable and erratic, it changed from moment to moment.

The next morning, I returned to Tracy's room in the ICU and found it transformed: Kelly, on one of the many, many trips she would make from Lincoln City, had brought a large scroll of white paper which she had covered with colorful photographs of Tracy's artwork and other photos that included him with friends he loved. She taped it up high on the wall so it was in Tracy's line of sight. In the coming days, more original artwork created by his friends showed up until the walls and the dreary window were covered in bright color denoting happy times on his beloved Oregon Coast. As the days went by, I found a small radio tuned to the local classical radio station and tucked next to the head of his bed; the scent of lavender; hand-dyed home-knit socks in Tracy's favorite colors wrapped in a green silk scarf scented with relaxing essential oils; a small healing blue Buddha; fresh flowers; a soft blanket across his bed; Heidi's intricately drawn and colored stars hanging from the wall – one had gone with Tracy on a trip to Europe and he had fun photographing it everywhere it went.

Frenetic energy bubbles out of Heidi, and it shows in her work that spans tiny, intricate dolls with moving parts to larger-than-life sculptural pieces as well as her fiercely protective love of animals in need. She and Tracy share a love of night skies and singing Pacific chorus frogs.

Tracy's Support for Tracy Facebook page had notes from those who visited, asking that other visitors bring something inspirational to read to him (but no cell phones because they interfered with the medical equipment) and for everyone to send him powerful healing and calming thoughts.

I spent five or six hours most days at the hospital during the 25 days Tracy stayed at OHSU. OHSU is a major Oregon employer, having a projected annual operating budget of $2.2 billion and employing 14,616 doctors, nurses, therapists, technicians, support and administrative staff. In 2014, capital expenditures were $218.8 million, and the Oregon legislature voted to invest another $200 million to support expansion of the OHSU Knight Cancer Institute. OHSU is a nationally prominent research university and Oregon's only public academic health center. Total patient visits in 2014 were 987,098; of that number, 22,061 were adults admitted for hospitalization; one-half of the hospitalized patients were insured via public payer or were uninsured.

Every time I left the hospital, I'd go home and hop on the computer with my list of new words: cerebellum, ischemic, hemorrhagic vs. clotting stroke. I looked for a brain "map" until I found one. I read and re-read the pamphlets and fact sheets from the American Heart Association and The American Stroke Association, which were provided by OHSU. OHSU takes medical education pretty seriously – including the education of people around those who suffer major health "events." Friends offered books and articles and websites to check online. The personal stories offered by so many served to connect all of us.

I was living on adrenaline, finding an internal drive even I didn't know I had. My life pattern had been to see what I could do to help others. My mother, a woman of immense personality, assessed the potential she saw in me very early in my life and made sure I understood two things: No one was going to wait on me and, since I had no particular beauty or talent, I should get used to working hard. If someone offered me something, I should be grateful and take it. I decided I wanted to learn how to make others' lives better. I discovered I was fascinated by how humans behaved and why. I felt safest staying in the background and observing. But, to make my life more complex, I also felt compelled to go a frightening step further -- to interpret, explain, offer reasons for other peoples' behavior, and try to make interpersonal relations work. I seem doomed to try to get bulldogs to kiss and make up. There are few challenges I won't take on, especially if I conclude that they might make someone's life better. From what I observed as a child, I assessed life to be hard, unpredictable and fickle. I have since added irrational, fragile and humorous to the list. I left my childhood when I was ten, when my sister died. I determined then that adults, not children, could make things happen. I believed that, as an adult if I worked hard enough at something, I could make it work. On the downside, I'm still trying to master the art of playing.

Why was I spending every waking hour trying to be at the hospital with Tracy? Why was I so focused on trying to learn all I could? Because I was terrified: Terrified he wouldn't make it; terrified that I might miss something I could do to make "The Difference;" terrified that someone who was supposed to be making him better would miss a step if I wasn't close by. Being terrified turned into a certainty: nothing worse could happen to Tracy as long as I was physically there to prevent it. In moments of greater rationality, I realized I was going a bit overboard, but I couldn't help it. I could *think* rationally, but I couldn't *feel* rationally. I believed Tracy had to have an advocate who was as close to being "always there" as possible. Who else would it be? He was unmarried and had no children. Born when my parents were 41-years-old, he was my only brother; I was his only sister. We always had been close.

When I learned something, I had an explosion of further questions. As I delved deeper into this "hemorrhagic stroke in the cerebellar region," I became increasingly frightened for my brother's future. I learned that hemorrhagic strokes differ from ischemic (clotting) strokes in several ways: the fatality rate is higher, and overall prognosis is poorer. One article indicated that 75 per cent of those who suffer a hemorrhagic stroke die within a few hours. Well, so far, he'd escaped that. I also found that people who have hemorrhagic strokes are younger; symptoms usually appear suddenly and this kind of stroke is often associated with a very severe headache, nausea and vomiting. Almost all of these disparate conditions appeared to be true.

In conversations with staff, I found myself trying to put the best face on the situation: "He's young to have had such a terrible stroke. He's in great shape. He has a great attitude about Life." The response was uniform: "Those are all plusses. But remember, it will be a long haul. He has had a traumatic brain injury, the extent of which we do not yet know. He very well may not recover fully, but we can hope that he will be an exception, that his recovery will be swift and positive."

Although retired from regular day-to-day jobs, Bill and I had full and busy but independent lives. We enjoyed coming together at the end of a day to compare notes of what we'd been doing. I was an active volunteer in my community, and Bill had a pretty extensive daily routine of his own that included writing his second novel.

Years before, we worked together in Carson City, Nevada, where I managed a statewide jobs program and served in one of my many interim posts, agency personnel and training director. Bill became the agency's communications director and worked closely with the governor's office. Later, I followed him to Washington, D. C., where he had gone to work for Nevada's senior U.S. senator. I laughed about us being slow learners; most people go to Washington. D. C. for a two-week vacation. It took us 12 years to see and do everything we wanted. Early in our marriage, he had gone on active duty with the U.S. Army for almost seven months in Honduras. After that, he took a driving trip around the country (part of it spent with Tracy with a lot of fooling around in places like Montana when they were supposed to be hightailing it back to the east coast). Bill then took the next several months writing fulltime on his first novel. I worked at the U.S. Labor Department in Washington, D.C., and kept the home fires burning. With a bachelor's degree in journalism, Bill had worked as a news reporter and editor for several newspapers in the West. He'd moved into public relations and communications in the national arena after getting a master's degree in economics, but creative writing was in his blood. Once a writer, always a writer, following his set routine, he often spent days at a time at his computer. He also was an active community volunteer spending hours each week outside the house. We often chuckled at his unofficial family title: Social Director. He loved arranging dinners and getting tickets for plays, symphonies, and other cultural events. We had a full schedule. And, he still had twice a week physical therapy and other doctor's visits for his slowly healing knee. The day after Tracy's stroke, he came with me to OHSU. The next several days he was otherwise engaged. He said he had prior commitments and it didn't seem as if he needed to be in Tracy's room all the time.

Five days after the stroke, Tracy seemed better. When prodded several times to tell us his name, Tracy said in a mushy sort of way, "My name is Tracy." A miracle four-word sentence! The next day, he passed a basic swallow test: if you can't swallow, you can't eat or drink. That same evening, some of Tracy's wonderful musician friends played a gig in Lincoln City and donated their tips to help with upcoming expenses.

Lincoln City, Oregon, is a beautiful place midway along Oregon's coast and peopled by an eclectic mix of individuals. Longtime Oregon residents remember when this part of the coast was a string of tiny towns interspersed with dense, dark evergreen forests. This was before Lincoln City gobbled up the four smaller towns around it. Those who've lived in the area for awhile distinguish where they live by calling out Taft or Delake or Ocean Lake or Nelscott. Over time, artists of all sorts drifted together and have become close but loose colonies along the coast. Many are solitary individuals as art often requires, but they all seem supportive of each other's endeavors. The Lincoln City area is where Tracy went to see if he could be an artist instead of a teacher. He has said many times he cannot imagine how lucky he was to find this particular and unique group of friends, and he says he absolutely knows he would never find such a group again anywhere in the world. For their part, more than one of his friends called Tracy the glue that held their community together.

In the days and weeks to come, friends and relatives who couldn't come hold Tracy's hand in person sent love, gifts, and what money they could to help make his life easier. It was so appreciated.

Six days after his stroke, he received real food. It was all things he liked: scrambled eggs, cranberry juice and soft pears. He dabbled with them, eating very little, but it was a start. The intricacies of eating food appeared to be beyond him. He put on a good show, but getting all the moving parts together wasn't working. Coordinating the whole function of eating was overwhelming and exhausting: picking up food with a utensil, making his hand and fingers work, getting the food to his mouth, chewing and swallowing. He fell back asleep before he ate much. He still couldn't see much beyond the edge of his bed. It seemed hard for him to focus on things and people farther away. His blood sugar was high; his blood pressure remained high.

A week after Tracy's stroke, I was much changed. I had a laser-like focus on Tracy, what was happening to him; what else could we do for him? Bill still needed rides to physical therapy. Friends became taxis when I wasn't available. I gave him short shrift otherwise. He got better fast, but he was definitely on his own. I concluded that he should understand; he was watching what I was going through. He knew me well. At this point, we had been in each other's lives for 38 years. We came together first as friends because we liked each other, not because we needed each other. Bill knew my family well, also. He's known my son and daughter since they were 12 and ten-years-old, respectively, and my brother since he was 20; I've known his daughter since she was three-years-old. Both our fathers were long gone, so when Bill and I married (It took us seven years of living together before we both wanted to get married at the same time), Tracy walked down the aisle with me and my son served as Bill's best man.

Bill kept making plans to go to dinner and keeping up with our regular life and I kept wondering why. I think he believed that as long as we acted as if everything were normal, life would get back to being normal faster. My garden suffered: it had been pampered for years and now looked like a sad, abandoned puppy. Dear friends stepped in. Mary and Linda, great friends and gardeners who share my birth year so we are ladies of a "certain age," spent the summer watering my plants to keep them alive. They also made me pause for an afternoon or an evening in one of their gardens, just to recharge a bit. I paid no attention to meals and postponed or excused myself from any engagement I could avoid. I was trying either to finish or come to an appropriate stopping point for some of my community volunteer projects involving trails, a parks and recreation bond oversight committee, and local elections. I thought if I could just keep my momentum going, I could last until I could gracefully disengage.

I cannot do justice to the depth of care and love evinced by Tracy's friends at this time, so just as one example, I offer words written by Kelly:

"Tracy, yesterday I came to see you. I brought with me photos and made a poster of pictures of you, smiling in every one. I want the doctors and nurses to know what an amazing and beautiful soul you are! Yesterday you wiggled your toes for me and I asked you to do it again, and you did! I am so excited that you are responding and making progress, even if it is little by little. Your whole being has been through a profound change and we must have patience while your body and mind sort out a new way. We must all come to our own center, like the glass I work, falling on center, which is how I am thinking about what you are doing. Coming to center. There is no force involved. We must wait for you to find your own new way. This is very hard. I know you are coming to center and I will wait and be there while you are falling, as are all of your friends, here to support you, as you find your way. I must say, that I myself, am feeling very disoriented, searching to find balance without your presence here in Lincoln City. You are the light that keeps us going. You are the one who sees the color and the beauty. There is a huge space that you occupy in all our hearts and minds and we carry you with us with every step in your time of healing."

I held my breath as I read the messages left by Tracy's friends. I understood then, from what I read, that he held a unique place in their lives. I knew that Tracy had always held a special place in my own heart. My mother was not built to have children. And yet, when my little sister died after years of agony from brain cancer, my mother determined to have another child because she didn't want me left alone. My father asked if she was nuts. She said, "Probably." But 22 months after my sister died, my brother, John Tracy, was born, taking more than two days to arrive. I came to realize what a gift I had received, in part because my mom had worked so hard to get him here, and because he was just so much fun to have around. I have many random memories. On his first day of school, the teacher asked who wanted to go home for lunch. He decided that he did, even though that wasn't the original plan. He was five years old. In a precursor of his great navigational skills and later love of travel, he walked home from his school on 29th Avenue to our home on 13th Avenue across several side blocks, stopping to chat and enjoy a banana with a road construction crew on his way. He walked into the house a little after 2 p.m. saying he'd like lunch. Years later, I asked him if he remembered this episode. I was reminded of it when he and I took off from a train in Florence, Italy, during a scheduled hour-long stop to go back to a store he'd been to once across the Arno River. He wanted to purchase a green belt he'd seen. Bill looked at us as if we were crazy, but I had no doubt that Tracy could find his way. We scrambled through alleys, up stairs, over bridges, around back yards, across plazas and he found the tiny store with no trouble whatever. However, we needed to run to return to the train before it pulled out of the station. And, yes, he did recall the episode of walking home for lunch. He said he'd looked at the packed lunch and decided one at home was better, and besides, it was a sunny day much too nice to stay indoors.

After the early days when I had plumbed the depths of *what* and *why* of this event, I wanted to know about potential changes caused by his stroke. What were the things we should look for? I'd watch him seem to get better only to slide back the next day. Was there another shoe to drop? Was he going to be a vegetable? Paralyzed? Depressed? Speechless? What about his art? I'm so glad I didn't know what was in store. Because it was about to get worse.

Nine days after his stroke, Tracy was still sleeping a majority of the time. When I came to see him in the morning, I wiggled his foot to see if he'd come awake to say hello. He awoke, smiled and said, "Hi." Then he said several more words. They made no sense. Two words that he repeated several times were "glove box." He patted his stomach when he said the words. I'm pretty creative, but this had me stumped. I asked him if there was something important in the glove box of his car. He has a much-beloved older Toyota 4-Runner named "Luna" that has taken him on many fantastic journeys. He nodded his head "yes."

Several times while I was there that day, the doctors and staff came in to listen to his heart. According to the monitor, it was "erratic." The medical team wanted to figure out what was happening and they also wanted to move ahead, taking the drain from his brain in the next day or so. A few days earlier, the medical team had begun "challenging" the overflow drain – slowly raising its level so less fluid/blood drained out. The plan was that Tracy's body would take over and absorb the fluids draining from the brain. One of the jobs of the aforementioned ventricle is to handle this drainage, something it does in all our brains. Since it was still not fully "re-inflated," it was having trouble doing its job. The hope still was that it would spring back and all would be well. If it didn't, the medical team would have to surgically install a permanent shunt, and they preferred not to do that.

I was at an early evening community meeting when I received a call from the doctor saying they wanted permission to take an in-depth look at the back of his heart. It would involve putting him under anesthesia, but it was something they felt should be done now, not later. I agreed. It seemed that Tracy's heart was enlarged. It was his body's way of accommodating high blood pressure. The medical team was so concerned about bringing down his stubbornly high blood pressure, they were trying increasingly aggressive ways to reduce it. The result was an irregular heartbeat. Tracy has the biggest heart in the world, and his heart was struggling.

One of his many visitors was Faith. Her experienced hands and elbows gave Tracy much-needed relief from lying motionless in a bed for all this time. She never touched his head or neck. She's a top-rate massage therapist and she shared her expertise so others of us could perform some of her magic when we spent time with him. It's amazing what gently squeezing toes and rubbing a foot can do. Intuitively, we all understood that touching Tracy was imperative, whether he was awake or not. We held his hand, rubbed his feet; just laid an arm next to his; put a hand on his leg. Someone close to him was touching him whenever he had visitors.

Twelve days after his stroke, we visited and found him with his eyes open, at least part of the time. Per usual, we read to him updates or emails we had received about him on his Facebook page. We joked. He smiled. He could say short phrases, but slurred longer sentences. His blood pressure was still a problem. The doctor told us it was increasingly clear that the blood vessels in his heart, brain and kidneys apparently had suffered from the chronic high blood pressure, describing his arteries and veins as being "brittle, like straws." He wasn't sure how that problem would play out going forward, but it sure scared me. The medical team planned to do an ultrasound of his heart in the next day or so to get a handle on the pressure, irregular heart beat and for the first time, they mentioned "tiny blood clots" and "A-fib." He would be sedated for this procedure. On this day we noticed that he tired so easily. He was no longer eating solid food; he was having more trouble swallowing. It appeared that his swallowing control mechanism was indeed damaged during the stroke. He had been an inveterate water-drinker. Now one sip made him choke. They installed a feeding tube in his nose as a temporary measure since he was not getting enough nourishment. That should also help with his debilitating fatigue, we thought. They had hopes of stabilizing him enough in the next few days to move him to an acute care ward.

I had more homework. I just knew that if I became expert enough, something bad couldn't jump out of the woodwork, so I sought out answers to every question I had, and I had a bunch of questions. What about those clots? I thought he had had "just" a hemorrhagic stroke, not a clotting stroke. And, what's "Afib?" Subsequent tests indicated that Tracy had indeed suffered a series of small clotting strokes. Reducing his blood pressure caused the upper chamber of his heart, the Atria, to "flutter." Afib -- Atrial fibrillation -- is a quivering or irregular heartbeat (arrhythmia) that can lead to blood clots, stroke, heart failure and other heart-related complications. When either heart chamber is not beating regularly and strongly, the blood slows down and may pool in the heart ventricle. If that occurs, the risk of clotting increases. In Tracy's case, that fluttering set up small clots that traveled to his brain. He now had at least two additional damaged areas in his head, besides the cerebellum, that required attention. And what can happen with blood vessels that are brittle like straws? How can his brain, heart and kidneys do their work if the blood vessels can't function properly? I never considered that there was a "swallowing control mechanism." I found myself noticing how I swallowed. There are enough "what-if's" here to scare any person to death.

Robin, dear Robin (I always think of her name as Robin, dear Robin) organized a visiting schedule and pulled so many people together to go see Tracy. She went herself regularly. Robin is a Renaissance woman: writer, teacher, actress, poet, photographer, beautiful soul and former neighbor of Tracy's. Less than two weeks after his initial big stroke, and between two visits when she spent several hours quietly sitting with Tracy, she wrote the following piece:

"He feels released. A smooth sweep of cells slipping swiftly through space. Spooning the horizon. A soft, slow song streaming out endlessly to trace the curve of the earth."

"Tracy." He hears his name like the touch of fingers brushing the pulse of his wrist. Then gone.

"Tracy!" He hears her now. Her little-girl laughter follows him into the garden. She lands beside him like a kitten. They smile at the rows and boxes of plants. They lean down in the heat. Sun burns the back of their necks. His hands scoop away the rich, black earth to make tiny beds for the seeds and she sprinkles them like salt from a paper envelope. Small grains of grace. He brushes the soil over the seeds and tips the watering can to soak them. The galvanized metal is hot in his hand and the water seeping its way into the dirt is already warmed by an afternoon in the sun. Dirt cakes his fingers. He rinses them with the water and dries his hands on his jeans. In the next bed, he pulls strawberries off the plants for both of them. He watches the red juice dribble down her chin and reaches out to wipe it with his handkerchief. He listens to the mellow buzz of insects, the rustle of wind through the apple tree, a hummingbird's wings.

"Tracy." He hears his friends speak in sentences like strands of beaded bracelets sliding past each other at his wrists. He runs them through his fingers. Jewelry to take with him as he leaves. On a journey of the most gentle geometry. The joy of a world so round. So easy to slide off. His spine grows long and bends into the arc of a circle. He spreads out like water. Pain leaves him. And fear. He joins this rush of sweetness that flows past us all. Boundless. He feels his friends with him. He is not lost.

The delicate strings wrapped round his wrists break away. The beads of words spill off the strands and fall to the earth like seeds. They are whispers in the earth. Prayers to tether him to the ground.

"Tracy, stop.

Tracy, stay.

Tracy, try."

They are earthlings. They stand beside his bed like wooden stakes. They tell stories made of twine to twist round his limbs. To tie him to themselves. They trace the outline of his hands with their fingers. They hold him to earth. They plant him in their hearts. Tracy.

He feels the return of time. The tempo of his heart. The track of sunlight across a day. He falls to his hands and knees, reaching out to the rich, black earth. There is the tangled, green garden hose on the ground next to him. The snap of breaking twigs under his feet. He scoops up a handful of soil and turns it over, letting some of it blow away in the breeze as it falls to earth."

For me, this was one of the darkest and most frightening times of Tracy's illness. The first was immediately following his stroke when we all were just reacting to what happened. Tracy held on instinctively to life. I believe that two weeks after his stroke, his hold on life was more tenuous. I think he was deciding whether to stay or not. I realized Robin saw that after reading her Facebook post.

All this time, Tracy's niece, my daughter, Alison, came with me to visit Tracy. Every day. Tracy, Alison and I had taken a sweet trip to France four years prior, and Tracy was the one who had made it an unforgettable seven weeks that we shared. Now, we had settled into a routine. I picked up Alison on the way to OHSU and I took her home afterwards. It gave us time to consider what we wanted to accomplish that day and to process what we had learned as we drove home. Fortunately for me, Alison is much like me and understood exactly what I was doing. Unfortunately, she is much like me and was driving herself mad (as I was doing myself) trying to control a totally uncontrollable situation.

Two weeks after Tracy's "event," I once again played bridge with my friends at our regular Monday afternoon game. I was to discover that this group of Bridge Sisters was my lifeline to sanity and survival. My Sisters loved me, cared for me, made me laugh after I made them cry, fed me, hugged me, gave me perspective by talking about their own loves and loved ones, and never let me win just because they felt sorry for me. Mondays were the days I looked forward to and they kept me going the rest of the week…and for the years to come.

Chapter 3:
Where are His Paintings?

Images of Tracy's paintings had been floating around the edges of my mind beginning a few days after he arrived at OHSU. Tracy is an artist. A gift from both our parents, but primarily our mother, his ability to record his images of the world around him as well as the ones in his head has landed his work in art galleries, offices, a hotel and homes around the world. His heart and eye always sought beauty and perfection in the world around him, often noting how it fell short of the ideal, and how to express what he saw.

After high school, Tracy worked in retail sales and was good at it. He then opened his own retail camera shop. People loved him but the business failed. He worked awhile for Nikon, traveling a lot and showing off the newest gadgets to photographers. It was fast-paced and exciting, but it left little time for any other life, much less time to create his own photographs. He has lived in places he loves and places he didn't like, and he discovered that "place" mattered so much to him he notably felt less well, less happy and less creative in places for which he had no affinity. I recall a camping trip where Bill, Tracy and I huddled out of the rain in a damp tent at Frog Lake on Mount Hood talking about what Tracy wanted to do with his life. Bill and I thought he seemed to be treading water, and asked what he really wanted to accomplish besides work in the K-Mart photo department.

Tracy said he'd love to be a photographer and artist, and to share how he saw the world by teaching. Bill asked why he didn't go to college. Getting a college education was always a "big deal" for both of us. Our parents didn't get to go, but Bill and I realized its benefits. It took me seven years to capture a bachelor of arts degree, and another year to complete my master's in guidance and counseling. In that time, I became a mother and discovered how much I needed college to allow me to provide any sort of life for myself and my children.

Reading had always been difficult for Tracy. In his experience, school was made up primarily of reading, so he hadn't been excited about pursuing more difficulty that, in his mind, got him no closer to art than he was already. We encouraged him to try college: it would be very different from high school.

As I sat in the waiting room, trying not to worry, images of Tracy's paintings pounced. Cascades of paintings full of color and horizontal lines washed over me like a tidal wave. Then the questions began. How many paintings does he have? Where are they? What's his inventory? How many galleries does he show in? Does anyone owe him money? Does he have any shows he's preparing for or any clients for whom he's painting on commission?

In large part, Tracy's paintings are Tracy. Always an artist, Tracy is both a professional photographer with a superb eye for black-and-white images and an "oil-on-canvas" painter. Beginning with a camera at a very early age, he recorded everything he saw around him. As a high-school freshman, he became the school sports photographer for the local newspaper. He wandered around the parapets and upper structures over the basketball court to get the shots he wanted until a teacher realized what he was doing and freaked out. One body of work he created juxtaposed the action of basketball with ballet; the commonality of the photos in this work showed the grace of movement in the air. His photographs often sought out the tiniest details at the same time they captured motion.

Later, Tracy crossed over to painting by drawing on his photographs. His paintings are large, colorful, abstract and three-dimensional. He loved the smell of oil and that he could mix his own colors. He moved to the Pacific Coast to determine whether he would like it. That was more than a dozen years ago. He expanded his creative repertoire to include using acrylic paint on various surfaces in part because it can take forever for paint to dry on the Oregon Coast. He might use a paintbrush -- he has some that are well-used -- so apparently he does. However, his usual method of applying paint is with a palette knife as he stands in front of a very large easel bolted to the wall that holds several of his large works-in-progress. He layers paint, and each layer requires drying time; thus he works on several pieces at once. One of the reasons he and Faith, his masseuse, know each other is that she is so good at assuaging the kinks in his shoulders, neck and back spurred by his painting style.

So, I began the hunt for Tracy's artwork. I realized I would need to go to

Lincoln City to his house and studio as soon as I could, but I didn't want to leave just yet. What if something awful happened when I was gone? I lectured myself: I knew a lot about his work, so if I just settled down and thought about it, I'd come up with at least some answers right here at home. If I would just let myself breathe, I'd be a lot better off.

When I returned home, I went to Tracy's website. It was a great history of past work and its status or location, but nothing current seemed to be there. I recalled he planned to re-work his website, but obviously he hadn't done that yet. I didn't have his computer passwords, so I would have to wait on any other access. I knew he painted in a studio at home and that he was working in a storefront studio on Highway 101 in Lincoln City, but I didn't know what work was in either place. He also was doing photographic work at his home studio, including poster-sized enlargements using a big commercial printer, and he had told me he was scanning a lot of old negatives and organizing them on his computer, but I didn't know the status of that project, either.

I thought about galleries. Where was he showing? I came up with five: two in Portland, one in Salem, one on the North Oregon Coast and one in Lincoln City. I needed to contact them. Again, I needed access to his computer for contact information. As I saw his friends, I asked them what they knew. He'd been working at the Volta Glass Gallery to make ends meet over the winter, so Kelly, who shows her glass work at Volta, and I discussed replacing him since they were going into their busy summer tourist season. I discovered he had a few pieces hanging there, as well. So that was six places he was showing various artwork.

Ten days after Tracy's "event," I drove to Lincoln City. I would be there six times before the fall season settled in. On this trip, I intended to check on his house and studios, see if I could access his computer, look for his previous year's taxes (they might give me a clue where to look for sales) and any other paperwork that might indicate what he had been working on when he left home that fateful afternoon to go to the gym. Since no one was at the house, I was concerned about leaving anything of value and wanted to check the locks to verify they could withstand any attempted break-in. I also wanted to check the glove box of his Toyota 4-Runner to see what was in there that was so important to Tracy.

Kelly met me at his house to give me the keys. I pulled up in front of his darling little house that looked so much like many other older little Oregon coast cottages. Kelly and I hugged and went into Tracy's house. I carried my overnighter into Tracy's bedroom and came back out into the living room. Kelly was sitting in a chair with tears running down her face. She said she was having such a terrible time trying to remain focused without Tracy there as her rudder. She said many of his friends expressed the same feeling of drifting. I felt like I was swimming upstream myself. She said she'd been in touch via email with Tracy's landlord. Tracy's rent was automatically paid from his credit union checking account and it had just been paid for the next month. So at least we had a month to figure out what came next. I told Kelly I wanted to look around and get an idea of what I needed to do right away. I also wanted to clarify the status of his studio on Highway 101.

Matt came by to see how he could help. Matt, who currently manages the local Pendleton Store in the Outlet Mall in Lincoln City, has been a close friend of Tracy's since Tracy first moved to Lincoln City years ago. Matt and his friend, Roger, took down the studio on Highway 101, packed it up and brought most of it to Tracy's house. On my next trip to the Coast, I helped move the paintings. I was impressed by the strength of the fabled coastal winds as I carried several of the bigger paintings outside to my car or their truck: the word "sail" did come to mind. The wind and the canvasses moved me around pretty good! Matt and Roger dismantled the overhead lighting system that Tracy built in the studio, took up the rug, and cleaned out the studio, bringing many big boxes heavy with paint and mineral spirits, oils, tints, bags of clean and used rags, brushes and palette knives, and a sound system back to his house. At the house, they put everything, except the paintings, in the room behind his garage. The paintings were the latest ones in a series that Tracy was working on, and they stacked them against the wall in the living room. Later, I repacked the boxes in the back room and moved them around because I needed the space to maneuver.

Matt and Roger took Tracy's pink "viewing chair," three worktables and the lighting system to Robin's garage. Robin, Tracy's Renaissance friend and former neighbor, had offered a large space in her garage to help store Tracy's things. The pink "viewing chair" had one prosthetic foot: a 4"x4" chunk of cedar acting as a foot replacing one that somehow had gotten lost years before. Tracy loved sitting in that chair which he placed in the center of the room several feet back from his easel in order to view his work-in-progress.

After Kelly left, I wandered all over Tracy's house that first afternoon. I opened cupboard doors and looked under the sinks. I opened the refrigerator (oops). I noted where he had paintings. In the house, many were hung, but I discovered at least a dozen of them in the room behind his garage that served as part unheated studio and part storage. It was a substantially sized room with not great lighting that seemed to stretch into the gloom clear back to the rear lot line. There were many paintings. In some cases, it was like greeting old friends because I hadn't seen them in awhile. I looked around guiltily to see if anyone was watching. Obviously, that was stupid, but I didn't want anyone else to see what I did. Tracy always let me touch his paintings. They are so structural with big overhangs and swirls of paint showing bare hints of other levels under the top layers of line and color. My fingers barely grazed the paint, tracing his lines across the canvas.

Abstract art depends a lot on the viewer. To me, some of his paintings breathe fire; some sizzle and blow my hair back like the wind; some undulate and swarm; some sing, but they all make me smile. Some paintings were ones he wanted to keep for himself. Some of the paintings were stacked vertically; some were in a section of the garage that I would term the hospital, because they needed to be doctored up based on dings from being moved around. Two very large paintings rested against an old, unused, refrigerator near the back of the room (which when I was eventually able to get the door open, I discovered housed very large pieces of what looked like a lighting system. For some reason, knowing Tracy, I wasn't at all surprised to find a lighting system in the refrigerator.) The paintings were so big, I was unable to move them except by using a corner of the frame as a pivot to see what else was behind them. Other paintings were rolled up out of their frames and there were many of those, too.

And then there were the photographic prints: hundreds of them, generally large, but some small. My memory whisked me back to a time at our dining room table when Tracy was about twelve years old. Dad had lived in Reno for a few years by then, and when I finished college, I moved there, too. Dad and Tracy were having a spirited discussion about F-stops. They had spent the day photographing at the cemetery in Virginia City. In those days before decent instant photographic results were possible, they were stumping for their favorite choices of speed and lighting. Mom looked at me and asked, "Where does an alien go to register?" Back in the present, I noted that some of the photographs were boxed and sorted and numbered in a mysterious system that I was sure made sense to Tracy. I found boxes and boxes of photographic paper in large boxes. I found an entire six-drawer wide console full of prints. I had never considered how heavy photographs are. This lesson was about to be reinforced when I went upstairs.

On the second floor, along one side of the steep stairs, there was a table made of a door resting on old IKEA legs. On top of that was a major project in process. It looked like maybe it would become a photography book, but now it was in several pieces along with long metal rulers, tissue paper, notes on different pieces of paper, and various photographs in no apparent order to a non-artist like myself. Under the table were boxes of prints, more photographic paper, and rolls of what looked like upscale butcher paper. In the one-bedroom upstairs was his two-hundred-twenty-five-pound commercial printer. I asked him once how he got it up there and he said, "With difficulty!" It appeared that he used a summer office upstairs. I guessed that in the cold of winter, he used just the downstairs area and shut off the upstairs. On the other side of the stairs on the second floor were several very heavy boxes that, upon examination, were full of photographic negatives, old prints, older cameras, and upwards of fifty journals full of sketches and ideas that Tracy kept through the years. The storage boxes were marked "No Wet!" in red thick-lined Sharpie, which explained why the heaviest boxes in creation were up a very narrow set of stairs on the top floor of his house that sits next to a creek at sea level on a part of the Oregon Coast that regularly practices tsunami drills.

I found Luna, his 1996 Toyota 4-Runner, backed into the garage, locked. Matt had driven her home from the gym and parked her so that if she wasn't driven for awhile and needed a battery charge, it would be easy to do. I would never have thought of that. We are a family that names its cars. Tracy's 4-Runner is Luna: the Spanish word for moon. One moonlit night, Tracy was looking at the Milky Way out the great moonroof that Luna offers and he decided to call his vehicle "Luna."

Harry was at the house that day, and he and I got into the car. I opened the passenger side, got in and looked in the glove box. We found registration and insurance papers; maps; some auto maintenance records; and a switchblade knife. We next checked the console. It had gloves, dark glasses, and some electronic cords. There were also a few CDs. I even checked the back storage area of the SUV, where Tracy had built several shelves that he used to transport paintings. I found nothing that I would consider of great importance to Tracy, so I was stumped. What did he think was in there?

When I went to bed that night, it was the first time I'd stayed the night alone in Tracy's house. When I visited previously, he always slept on a blow-up mattress in his office, insisting I take his bed. This time, I felt so very alone. Even Bill wasn't here. I climbed into the bed, purposely not changing sheets just so I could smell Tracy. I plunged my face into his pillow, took a deep breath and came out sobbing. I cried a long time. Since I couldn't do anything else right then, that was probably a good thing. My eyes were puffy and my nose stuffy the next morning, but so what? My brain was a little clearer. I don't do well crying in front of other people, so through the summer as I was given little windows of opportunity, that's when I cried – and later, yelled all the epithets and foul language I know. As I drove back-and-forth, to-and-from, Lincoln City, I played CDs of operas, turned up the volume and more than once, just yelled over the sopranos. Friends asked how I looked so calm. I answered that they weren't riding in the car with me as I drove to-and-from Lincoln City.

As I took another look around Tracy's house and storage area the next morning, I noted stacks of wood for frames, new canvas and boxes of paper, some opened, some not. It appeared that Tracy recently had received a shipment of materials. I hunted around in the boxes and came up with a shipping list. Based on that, I found most of the order – apparently he already had constructed a few frames and used some of the photographic paper – but I never found everything. Kelly called the supplier, explained the situation, and the supplier said if we could match framing material by size to its shipping container and shipping list, the company would take everything back. I contacted Tracy's friend, Jane, a fellow photographer with whom he had shared a studio in years past, and his friend, Sharon, a big fan of his work and of him. Sharon is a highly skilled and creative chef, teacher, and a born sales person. She never let an opportunity slide if she thought she could get a potential buyer to pay attention to Tracy's work. She still has one of his bigger works hanging above the teaching/demonstration area at the Lincoln City Culinary Center. (So that's seven places I knew his work was hanging.) She always says she loves it, but she also tells her audience of folks taking culinary classes at the Center if anyone sitting around the demonstration area wants to buy it, they can have it right now. Jane and Sharon helped sort out where to begin with his paintings and his photographs. We decided to get the return order of photographic supplies together which meant finding and matching items with the shipping list, matching each box with its routing number, boxing, putting an inventory list in each box, re-taping, and addressing several boxes. This consumed many days.

Sharon went with me to one local gallery, where we knew Tracy had work hung, but we didn't know specifically which pieces. I was concerned because, as far as I knew, the corporate headquarters of that gallery still owed Tracy money from several years before, and I didn't want to leave work there unattended. Tracy is a very quiet, polite partner when it comes to his galleries. But he is also a hands-on manager: he was in touch with all his galleries on a frequent and regular basis. I knew I must protect his work and his financial interests. When Sharon and I visited the gallery, she wandered around trying to spot Tracy's paintings. I talked with the local sales person, a genuine fan of Tracy's work who expressed his shock at what had happened to Tracy. It's a small community; everyone knew. I told him I was frankly concerned about leaving Tracy's paintings there – not because of him – but because of the current state of accounting and the fact that the company still owed Tracy money for paintings previously sold. He gave me contact information and said if I wished to take the paintings, he understood. I asked him to give Sharon a complete list of the paintings over the next couple of days. He said he would wrap the paintings and make them ready for pick up. He was a total gentleman caught in a very uncomfortable situation.

While still at Tracy's house, I went through files, drawers and boxes until I found an old set of files indicating which paintings the gallery still owed him for payment. I took that file with me and subsequently contacted the gallery's accountant. We met several times to reconcile what I had found in Tracy's records and what information the accountant had. We came to an agreement. The gallery sent a check later in the year for one of the four paintings, agreeing they still owed for; a second check for another painting was received a year later. It took them another two years to pay him for the two most expensive paintings they sold, for which they had collected the payments, but never paid Tracy. I am happy to say that this difficulty was unique to this one gallery Tracy did business with.

I left Lincoln City for home a day and a half later, leaving big requests with his friends. I didn't know what else to do but ask. They all have jobs and kids and families and health issues and more… just like everyone, so I knew that anything I asked was an imposition. Without exception, they gracefully took on whatever I asked and offered to do more.

Over the next six weeks, Sharon and I created, and then many times modified, a comprehensive list of Tracy's paintings. We started with the ones in his house and studio. We itemized them by where they were located and whether they were completed (as in ready to sell); incomplete new work; or work that was in Tracy's personal collection and thus not for sale. He always put one painting aside from any series he completed. I asked him once if it was the prettiest or nicest or biggest or in his opinion the best of the series. I loved his answer. He said he always kept aside the one that *taught* him the most.

I asked Harry, a very recent high-school graduate who had set up the "Support for Tracy" Facebook page, to come to Tracy's house and make sense of Tracy's computer system because I needed to know where all his paintings were located, contact information for galleries, and the status of his paintings. For example, some paintings were rented out for six-month terms; others were sold and the galleries were collecting time payments. People began asking me what was available for sale. They wanted to purchase some of Tracy's work. I put them off. I didn't know enough. Harry found sufficient information so I could contact galleries when I got back to my home in Beaverton.

By that point, Tracy's newest paintings were in his living room. Several different sizes, they had uniquely shaped trees in them along with his signature horizontal lines. Their intensity was pastel, something unusual for Tracy. To my untrained eye, they were delicate, intricate, with smaller details than had appeared in earlier work. I don't recall if all were unsigned. I spotted a tiny painting just 6 3/4"x 8," and was concerned that in all the hubbub of moving it might get either lost or damaged. I took it home with me. Tracy knows I have it. When he's ready for it, I'll return it, but for now, I drink it in on a daily basis.

I was able to go back-and-forth to Tracy's world in Lincoln City because Bill and Alison took care of things at home for me when I was gone. So focused was I looking at life through my lens, I assumed Bill saw everything the same way. As I thought about things over time, I realized there were severe differences. While my early life was spent with a tight-knit loving family, Bill's growing-up time was spent in difficulty, uncertainty and trauma. Like his older sister, he couldn't wait to get away from home. He began trying to leave while in the seventh grade after his mother attempted suicide, lied to get into Air Force boot camp at age 16, and left for good at 18 years old. He made his own life, beholden to no one. In the course of time, he married, divorced, married and then divorced twice the mother of his only daughter, and then lived with me for several years before we decided we might as well get married. He had a series of stepfathers after his father died of carbon-monoxide poisoning in a closed garage, with a little help from alcohol, when Bill was twelve years old. Bill hadn't had much experience feeling loved and cared for – or in loving and caring for someone else. He knew early on in his life if he was going to be anything, he had to do it himself. He didn't lean on anyone. He shares with me but not comfortably with others. He doesn't want anyone other than himself to be in control of his life, and he doesn't want to be responsible for other people. He told me when we first met at work in our early thirties, that he loved that I was independent. He didn't want someone who would lean on him or smother him. Mentally, he understood that I loved Tracy and would care for him forever, if need be. Emotionally, that engulfed him in claustrophobic terror – and not a little anger. His life had been changed by external circumstances over which he had no control. He had worked very hard to run his own life, looking toward the time when his life would be his own to enjoy every day. I came to understand that the reason Bill didn't leave was because he loves me more completely than he loves anyone else. He didn't plan it that way, it just is. He greatly cares for and admires his daughter and loves his grandchildren, and he cares for my family and his brother and sister, but me, he just plain loves, no matter what. He does anything in his power he thinks will make me happy. Just like me, he can't help who he unreservedly loves.

A week later, I was back in Lincoln City for a day. I walked into Tracy's house and found the refrigerator grossly fragrant; mail, generally junk, stuffed the mail box; the boxes of materials still not shipped. Sharon had matched all the numbers and sizes she could, but some just did not match. She had made notes and left them on the coffee table in the living room. After wandering through Tracy's house the week before, I had decided to sort his paintings into different rooms: the ones available for sale in the living room; the newest ones and those not for sale in Tracy's collection in his bedroom. I counted more than seventy paintings plus four three-dimensional sculptures several feet tall, but not including the ones off their frames. There were also other framed pieces: some were his photographs; some were created by other artists. He sometimes traded pieces with other artists. Since he had photographs and photographic paper in several places, upstairs and down, I decided to consolidate them in the garage. I hoped any upcoming tsunami would wait until we moved his art to a safer place.

A week later, I was back in Lincoln City. As before, I parked in front of his house. I checked the mailbox and Kelly's efforts to pick up his mail were evident: there were just a few pieces. I found the rest inside. I walked through the little gate in the white picket fence around the yard, noting that flowers were blooming in total abundance and abandon, and sat my overnighter down in the little vestibule while I got the key and opened the door. I was hit by a double whammy: the house was totally silent, unlike when Bill and I visited Tracy before when there was always music, and it smelled so much of Tracy's things. I got inside and shut the door before I sank down on the floor and sobbed. His house was waiting for him, but it had been left alone unexpectedly for a long time. I quit blubbering, got up, put my stuff in his bedroom, and went to the kitchen to get a drink of water. The faucet still leaked. He'd tried to get it fixed months ago. I tweaked it until it mostly shut off.

Sharon and I went back to the gallery in town, picked up his paintings and brought them to Tracy's home. Adding those and the ones we took from his studio on Highway 101, there were more than one-hundred paintings at his house. Sharon and I were trying to see what was available for sale. At this point, Tracy had no medical insurance and hadn't been approved for Medicaid/Oregon Health Plan. His medical bills already were astronomical. His paintings were all he had.

We continued to update the inventory of paintings after I talked with representatives of Tracy's galleries. All wanted to help. They also schooled me in the art/gallery/painting world. I learned about how art is rotated in and out of a gallery, how to discern what the gallery is looking for in new or other work new to them, how to represent Tracy at openings or shows (I negotiated with the gallery representatives: they talked about his work and I talked about Tracy. I had no idea how to present his work! I just loved it, that's all). I learned that selling in the art world, like sales anywhere, is competitive. Negotiating with one gallery representative who has a client and another who has a desired painting was interesting. Bill and I learned how to pick up and deliver paintings. On the same weekend that we were moving Tracy out of his house, a dealer came to the Coast to see if there were some paintings she wanted for her gallery in Salem. She saw how we had stacked and stored the paintings, having just put them into the storage unit earlier that morning. Alison and I thought we had done a good job of separating and padding each one, but the dealer showed us how to do it right, with the proper materials.

She also took away six paintings, all in the back of her cute little VW Beetle. Later she discovered damage to one of the paintings. She said she could try to sell it at a discount, but I didn't want any defective or imperfect paintings out there. Tracy wouldn't do business that way. In just another example of nice people doing nice things just because they can, she contacted another artist who had exchanged work with Tracy, and he offered to fix it.

Matching the actual paintings to the list was always a challenge. I kept finding paintings that had no presence on any computer list or website. Friends would tell me they knew there was a "Tracy Painting" hanging in other places: the coffee shop, a restaurant, the Glass Gallery. Discoveries like this just added to the puzzle: were those paintings for sale or owned by the business or on display and not for sale? I checked gallery websites where Tracy had work. Some paintings were listed on one gallery's website, but in the records I could find, the paintings were somewhere else. Trying to find where the real painting was, as opposed to where it was listed on a piece of paper was quite a game. I also found names but could find no paintings. Some had changed names because, I discovered later, Tracy would decide to paint over an old one that he, for some reason, didn't like. Later, when I complained to Tracy about never coming up with a clean and complete match of paintings and inventory list, he laughed. He had more than eight-hundred paintings to his credit, and he knew where every single one was. Since the "master list" was in his head, and his head was otherwise engaged at this point, I was chasing down any clue I could find.

When we moved Tracy's paintings available for sale to a climatized storage unit in mid-August, we were still trying to discern Tracy's wishes for each painting. Early on after his "event," we could tell that Tracy knew his paintings. He hadn't forgotten them. Sometimes he had difficulty telling us their names and sometimes he didn't know exactly where they were, but he always knew their content and size. We began asking him about specific paintings: was it for sale or did he want to keep it? I was afraid of selling something he didn't want sold. We were concerned about the possibility that his existing paintings were the last he might do. With great luck and good fortune, perhaps he would again paint, but surely the work would be different. As time passed, Tracy also began to contemplate his paintings differently. He increased the not-for-sale list. So Sharon and I continued to adjust the inventory as things moved around to different galleries – and between the living room and back bedroom -- and Tracy rethought what he wanted to happen to his work. We wanted the pieces in the storage unit to be available for viewing if anyone was interested in purchasing them. We had checked with Tracy's website and a few paintings were not listed or pictured there, so we took pictures of each piece available for sale. Tracy, no doubt, had pictures of all his completed work, but I couldn't figure out where they were located.

We moved the rest of Tracy's paintings to another storage unit so they would not be confused with the ones for sale. On the day his friends moved them out, Jane, his photographer friend and former studio-mate, taped a note with a list of paintings on the glass in the door between the garage and the back storage unit of the house. It said, "I took these. Also – there is a garden snake in the garage so don't everyone freak out! And be careful with it (smiley face)." That's appropriate: In the Chinese calendar, Tracy is a Snake (as am I).

Before we moved the paintings from his house into the storage units, Bill put me in contact with a friend of his, an experienced insurance broker, because I thought we should insure Tracy's paintings. It was one thing for Tracy to decide to keep a close watch on his paintings when he was at home or in his studio rather than insuring them. It was another thing entirely to care for his work from afar. I got some more schooling, this time in the world of insurance. We settled on a Fine Arts Dealer policy. I just hoped nothing would go amiss because any painting I deemed "irreplaceable" meant that it was "uninsurable" precisely because it couldn't be replaced if Tracy never painted again. I also reviewed past tax files to try to figure how the paintings were valued. I learned that when sold, that established a value for that painting. For those not yet sold, their value, as far as the Internal Revenue Service was concerned, was the cost of materials that went into the paintings. Period. So much for lots of valuable paintings just waiting to be sold!

I came to realize that selling art was about as easy as selling a house during an economic downturn: lots of desire to purchase, but not lots of ability. It also became clear that while there are many artists and photographers in the world, very few actually make a living creating photographs and art. I was asked about selling his paintings at a discount, just to make some money. I decided not to. I did agree to sell his work through either his existing galleries or the Lincoln City Cultural Center and to take time payments for sales. There was never enough income to do much more than offset ongoing business expenses. His business needed him back.

While Tracy, Bill and I were settling into a routine in the Portland area, his friends gathered together on Tracy's behalf in mid-December, 2011 at Eden Hall in Lincoln City. It was a bitter-sweet time. In previous years, Tracy had invited his friends to Eden Hall for an evening of wine, cookies and hearing his latest "travelogue" with photos he'd taken in Italy, France, Germany, Switzerland, Slovenia, the Czech Republic and Hungary. As I looked around the Hall at one of those earlier evenings of fun, I realized that the Hall was full. Tracy had a myriad of friends! The dialogue back-and-forth at those gatherings reflected everyone's enjoyment that so much of the substance in his photographs showed up in his later paintings. He also took a lot of good-natured ribbing about his photographic focus in these beautiful places: his fetish with chairs and construction cones, for example. On this December occasion, friends hung several of Tracy's paintings and many of his photographs so old friends were reminded of his work and new friends were introduced to it. The mid-December event was by many measures a exceptional success. A major accomplishment, as they themselves noted, was that Tracy always was the one to bring them together and here he was, doing it again. Previously, he hosted Wine Fridays and here it was again, almost. It gave the artists an informal and lively venue to showcase their latest work for each other. Musicians made the night festive. It gave chefs and caterers a chance to offer their culinary delights to their friends to celebrate the season and the fact that Tracy was still on the planet to celebrate this year's holiday season. His friends used the time to write cards to Tracy. Later, once the dozens of cards were delivered to our house, he spent days going through them.

His friends, again led by Matt, Robin, and Sharon, pulled off another extravaganza a few months later with a month-long art show featuring several artists, including Tracy, in the PJ Chessman Gallery at the Lincoln City Cultural Center. Following the festive opening, which featured light refreshments and superb local musicians, his friends again took the opportunity to catch up on Tracy's condition and share their joy that, although he was on a long journey, he was "coming back." In a new and rather creative wrinkle, the Lincoln City Cultural Center acted as the gallery/broker for sales at the event, to the benefit of Tracy as well as other artists who sold their work during the show. It is a creative way for them to help artists. Tracy received income from them over several months as patrons made time payments for their new treasures.

For each of these events, Bill took paintings from Portland to the storage unit in Lincoln City, and Tracy's friends moved them in-and-out of the storage unit as they needed to for the shows. Without their commitment and care, neither the benefits nor the continuing public focus on Tracy and his work would have happened. Without his friends, I still would be chasing down paintings. When we talked about it all later, Tracy smiled and said he was so humbled that everyone went to such trouble for him. To this day, I don't know the details of why Tracy is so important to each of his many friends. I just know that they are tenacious in their allegiance and loyalty to him and say, generally, that he was there for them at some point when they needed a friend. I told him he owed them all: he had to get well enough to move home to them. They missed him so terribly.

Chapter 4:
What Goes On in an Acute Care Unit...

In the evening of the sixteenth day after Tracy's stroke, he moved to the Kohler Pavilion Acute Care Unit on the tenth floor of Oregon Health Sciences University Hospital. Much had happened in the last few days. Tracy hated the feeding tube, so they removed it when he promised to eat. Based on the struggles he had eating and drinking, everyone knew he would need encouragement. Other tubes were removed as well; things like the catheter. Staff had him up in a wheel chair. He was responding well to questions and doing what they asked him to do. Blood pressure remained stubbornly fickle. The view of Portland and the mountains is spectacular from the hallways around Tracy's room. I hoped he would get to enjoy them. He would be in this room for nine days.

It's a mystery to me as to what medical changes occurred to allow Tracy to move from Neurosciences ICU to the acute care unit. As a non-medical person, I saw several unresolved problems that didn't seem to have gotten any better between the time he was in the ICU and then the acute care unit. Don't get me wrong, the folks in the Acute Care Unit were as nice and professional and caring and attentive as the folks in the ICU. I just wondered why having unresolved high-blood pressure, a fluttering heart, high-blood sugar, trouble eating and drinking, exhaustion, damage from blood clots in his brain, in addition to the still unresolved injury caused by the hemorrhagic stroke were suddenly different from one day to the next. I concluded the key was *stability*. Things weren't resolved, but they were relatively stable: his blood pressure remained out of whack, sometimes low, sometimes high, but they knew it was out of whack. So, maybe that's the reason for moving. The Neurosciences ICU doesn't contain an unlimited number of beds. A friend suggested that maybe there had been a rash of accidents with head traumas and they needed the space for people even worse off than Tracy. Who knows?

All his pictures and banners, blankets, socks, and good luck charms came with him. Lyn, yet another artist friend from Lincoln City, put them up in his new room.

Bill came to visit when I specifically asked him to, just to be there if I couldn't be. As time went on, and daily changes in Tracy's behavior seemed minimal to him, he resisted regularly visiting. He didn't like his routine disrupted, and if there were to be disruptions, Bill preferred knowing about them ahead of time. He's a planner and an organizer and he doesn't like sudden changes in his plans especially when the changes are made by others. In fairness, he had taken over many of our regular household duties, and he put off two long-planned trips because he knew that I needed him. One day when I was not in town, Bill went to see Tracy with Alison. There was a bit of applesauce left in a cup on Tracy's tray. Bill offered him a spoon. Tracy is right-handed, and he took it with his right hand. Bill held the cup. Tracy needed help scraping out the cup, but he got the applesauce to his mouth (better by far than a week ago). He was less capable with his left hand. One of the clotting strokes caused weakness on the left side, but another caused difficulty with controlling fine motor skills in his right hand – the one he uses to paint. So he had challenges now with both hands. During the same visit, Alison held up a bouquet of flowers sent from a friend, and asked Tracy to tell her what color they were. He got it right: yellow.

During his stay in the acute care unit, we discovered more continuing challenges for Tracy and those around him. As he moved more, got out of bed more, stood up more, went to different areas of the hospital in a wheel chair, was visited by a different sort of staff – therapists – who asked more of him, we all began to notice evidence of wide-spread injury and damage. I can attest to how appalled I was at what I saw now with my used-to-be articulate, composed, organized, funny and accomplished little brother. I cannot imagine what this all must have looked like through his eyes.

Because of the type and location of his original stroke, he had trouble with fatigue and downright exhaustion; he had no balance; he was dizzy and nauseated all the time except when he could lie down and be very still. His senses seemed distorted or heightened. He jumped at loud noises. He preferred to stay in a room that was darker because bright light was physically painful. It seemed that his eyes were unable to regulate the amount of light entering them. I kept hoping we could take him to the outside viewing area that overlooked the city of Portland with Mt. Hood in the background. He was born in Hood River and the mountain was a daily presence for his first six years of life. He so loves the outdoors and he had not been there in ages. We never made it.

It became apparent that Tracy had lost some short-term memory capability. He didn't remember being told what had happened to him even though I, and several others, had told him various abbreviated versions. What was interesting though, was that he did remember that we had asked him to try to do everything his medical team asked of him. His blood pressure and his blood sugar continued to shoot all over the place. Upchucking was now a regular occurrence. He was vomiting many times a day. It was related to movement/balance, but it must have been awful for him. He was not getting much value from the food he ate because it didn't stay in him long enough. He was losing weight. Of course, we all, Tracy included, joked about his "food" -- a special soft diet of extruded carrots and some sort of soft taupe-colored soup, for example, because he had such difficulty swallowing. He had more difficulty with thin liquid like water than with this food.

Right about the time Tracy moved to the acute care unit, he was visited by friends Allan and Carol from Reno. Allan had known Tracy since they worked together in a pizza parlor in Reno after high school. Once, Allan made a mayonnaise pie for Tracy because Tracy made no secret of how he hated mayonnaise. Another time, they went camping together and, according to Tracy's story at the time, it was Allan's responsibility to bring the tent. He did, but he forgot the poles! Allan said he'd brought the tent: Tracy should be responsible for something. At one point in his life, Allan was successful in real-estate sales and was instrumental in getting his boss to hire our mother as a secretary after our dad died. As time went by, Allan was a tremendous help to me, and indirectly to Tracy, because I used him as a sounding board. Allan had gone on to earn a Ph.D in psychology. He understood the physical changes that had happened to Tracy and was able to deduce what the ramifications were and what the possible outcomes might be. He and Carol also brought two books that were incredibly helpful. They became dog-eared as I referred to them again and again: *"Living with Stroke, a guide for families"* by Richard C. Senelick, M.D. and *"My Stroke of Insight – A Brain Scientist's Personal Journey,"* by Jill Bolte Taylor, Ph.D. Allan and Carol also introduced me to TED TV, where I watched Jill Bolte Taylor speak about her experience. She had a stroke that left her pretty much speechless, and I was almost speechless as I listened to her. Much later, Tracy discovered TED TV on his own and was mesmerized by Taylor.

Dr. Senelick's *'Living With Stroke, a guide for families,'* isn't a large book but I read it like I suspect most of his readers do: searching the glossary for words that related to our specific situation to uncover what had occurred and what was important to know right now. I discovered that the location of a stroke is more important than how big it is. In high-school biology, my eyes glazed over trying to memorize the parts of the brain. I always confused cerebrum and cerebellum. This book set me straight. We all learn something when it matters to us. I learned that the cerebellum is what Dr. Senelick calls The Office Coordinator. "... Just behind the brain stem, and slightly above it, sits the cerebellum, a mass of tissue that coordinates our every movement. It helps us keep our balance, allowing us to hold a glass of water steady. The cerebellum also coordinates the movements of our speech muscles ..." Dr. Senelick later in the book noted "...the cerebellum, like the brain stem, controls many of our instinctive functions. It is here that reflex actions are born, where our balance and coordination find a center..." He listed various symptoms, and I ticked off every one of them as they related to Tracy: slurred speech, abnormal movements or tremors, ataxia (the lack of muscle coordination), imbalance, dizziness, queasiness and nausea, uncontrollable vomiting. Yup, every single one. And Tracy had some extras for good measure, for example, swallowing and choking, and incorrect reactions to sensory cues (smelling things that weren't there). That might be because his stroke apparently didn't recognize a strict boundary between cerebellum and brain stem. Dr. Senelick noted several brain stem stroke symptoms that also related to Tracy: impaired swallowing, a loss of balance caused by the brain stem's connection to the cerebellum, unstable blood pressure as well as nausea and vomiting. Doctors, as they later discussed Tracy's post-stroke actions, would slide around the stroke location, including both cerebellum and the brain stem in their evaluations. And, a few more problems presented themselves: left-side weakness and issues related to poor short- term memory, speech, word search and comprehension based on having had three other strokes in different areas.

The staff was trying to help Tracy with what I call the Triumvirate of Therapies (physical, occupational and speech) since he had been inactive for almost a month. They also wanted to evaluate how well he could transition from a bed to a wheel chair or walker as well as increasing his activity. Going forward was paramount. Staying static was a death knell. Late one morning, the physical therapist had Tracy sitting on the side of his bed, getting him ready to stand up and hang on to a walker. Tracy groaned, said something unintelligible and then passed out back onto the bed. His blood pressure had plummeted. Instead of taking a turn with a walker, he was in bed, clammy, pale, shaking and nauseated. There were ever so many of these turns for the worse. Through it all, he never gave up. He never said he didn't want to do what the physical therapist (PT) asked. The PT said he was rare: one who so wanted to get better. Tracy knew what was being asked of him and why. He went to all possible lengths to meet the hopes and prayers for him. Every day, he became a little brighter and a little more present in the moment. He taught us that while we all cheered his good days, we needed to understand how hard they were for him to manage. Some days would be very tough and they needed just as much cheering as the seemingly good ones did. But he positively never, ever gave up. How could we do any less?

Challenges and difficulties to overcome are sort of like operations -- mine is much harder/worse/tougher than yours because it happened to me. Timing is important too: Now gets much more attention than some other time. Thus from Tracy's very beginning on his road to recovery, he was more aware of what was being asked of him, in the immediate. On any scale of measurement, what had happened to Tracy was really, really bad. He couldn't hold a thought for long, but he clung to "getting better." Magically, a bad day was inevitably followed by a special gift: friends sending loving thoughts and visiting with gifts and tales of home.

One Facebook posting from Heidi, his sculptor friend who shares his love of night skies and Pacific chorus frogs, was: *"Thank you everyone, for all that you share here... it is so nourishing, comforting...wonderful...Tracy I love you...and I'm missing you a lot...I talked to you tonight, on the front porch, looking at the stars and listening to the frogs. I love you. Heidi."*

Other friends told him that what he was being asked to do was very hard, but that he needed to continue to try hard. He always said that he would. Cynthia, a friend who shares Tracy's love of the Earth's special places and wanders between Lincoln City and Hawaii, posted on Facebook...

"Tracy's spirit has not changed through all of this. He smiles every time he opens his eyes and lets you know that this thing will not beat him. He has such a great attitude and seems to care so much that people are concerned, even when the nurses talk sweetly to him and adjust his pillows, etc. I keep telling the nurses what a special person he is. I have a friend who was an ICU nurse for 30

49

years and she says this is important. So show your love and keep visiting and posting."

During a visit, Heidi (who, along with her husband, Dave, has rescued so many animals and given them a happy home on their farm) brought a 5" x 7" glossy picture of a special pig named *Madison*. This pig was spoon-fed at Heidi's, and Tracy knew *Madison* well. Tracy reacted to the photograph by talking in his special "*Madison* voice," which he shared with Heidi. (Later, Heidi would tape a tiny picture of *Madison* to the railing of Tracy's bed, right where he could see it. She and Tracy tried to convince a nurse that Tracy slept with *Madison* at home. The nurse didn't buy it.) Heidi's conclusion after a "wonderful time" visiting Tracy was *"...Tracy you are doing so incredibly well!!! In one week's time, you have made so many strides... We're doing it Tracy... You're doing it... you will and you are. I love you to the moon and back a million, million times."*

Friends from a lifetime ago (the Magical Summer of 1984 at Camp Orkila on an island north of Seattle with a bunch of kids and grownups, supposed camp counselors who were also kids) talked of "those great times" and asked that we mention the coordinates D5 on a West Virginia road map to him. I did. It drew the laugh they were hoping for.

I've heard that you can judge a person by the friends he keeps, and even more by the long-time friends he keeps. If that's the criteria, Tracy must be near the top of the list of good people. He has an amazing array of friends scattered everywhere. The content of what Robin, Renaissance woman, posted on Facebook is a perfect example of his affect on people.

"Dear, dear, Tracy, Usually I don't write much here. I read what others say and "like" their words. But the past two Mondays I have been in Portland with you, and today I will not be there. So I find myself missing you more than usual this morning. And if I can't talk to you (especially now that I hear you are talking back!) I must at least write.

It's fun how, even though you aren't here, I sometimes think I see you. I see you walking around Taft [a small community within Lincoln City] or driving down the street. A few days ago, I saw a bright yellow kayak in Schooner Creek and thought to myself, "Good for Tracy – he's out enjoying the sun and the water." I drive by your studio and still crane my neck – the way I have always done when I drive by your studio – to see if you are working and to catch a glimpse of you painting. In the morning, when I'm sitting down at Pacific Grind with a latte, I expect you to walk in the door at any moment. I turn around every time someone comes through the door, knowing that your face will be the next face I see. And you will be smiling. And you will sit down in the cozy chair with your iPad in your lap and your coffee sitting on the arm of the chair or on the little white bookshelf to the left. But you will ignore your iPad and I will ignore the book sitting on the table in front of me and we will talk. You will talk in a thousand different directions at once, looping in circles back and back again, shooting off on tangents with your eyes sparkling. And I will laugh at you because you always make me laugh with your conversational "style" and you will laugh too because that is what you do.

"These times when I think I see you, or when I expect to see you, always make me smile. Because they remind me how much you belong to us. How you are always in the right place when you are here with us. How we here all hold a part of you with us each day. I am aware now, like I never was before, how many little things happen during the day, during the week, and I say to myself "I'll save that for Tracy... I've got to tell Tracy about that... ask Tracy about that... get Tracy's opinion about that... share that with Tracy because he'll smile about that..." Right now, you are like the last piece of the puzzle that is so essential, and we are all just waiting to have you back here with us, so you can make the picture exactly right, perfectly complete, with your color, and the way that you fit here with all of us who are missing you patiently, but every day. And we are holding your place for you like a puzzle piece in our hands. So come back as soon as you can, Tracy. Because we are waiting."

Now the medical team was saying that as soon as they thought his physical condition was stable, and there was a post-OHSU place for him to go, he would be moving. I looked around and discovered it was my job to find that facility. I enlisted Bill's help. Our intent was to find a short-term location that would offer therapy and time to gain strength so he could get into "Rehab Boot Camp" in the next two months. Rehabilitation Institute of Oregon (RIO) in Portland was the center we were aiming for because it had a reputation of real, intense and swift improvement for people like Tracy, who had suffered traumatic brain injury. Rather than serving as the end of the line for people with traumatic brain injury, RIO creates personalized patient plans that include goals and a target date for discharge. RIO, located at Legacy Good Samaritan Hospital and Medical Center in Portland, is an acute inpatient care facility providing high-intensity rehabilitation therapy and counseling as well as medical services around the clock. Aimed at enabling participants to return to living in the community following strokes and other conditions producing significant disability, RIO treats more than 500 patients a year, with about 92 per cent returning to live successfully in the community. The national average is 77 percent. RIO also has better long-term results than those treated at a skilled nursing home. Time was of the essence, if everything we read and heard from professionals was right: the best and greatest recovery after a stroke comes in the first six months. After that, much of the "common consensus" was that wherever a stroke victim had progressed at six months was pretty much where he/she was going to stay. In time, the dichotomy between the medical profession and insurance providers/caseworkers became more apparent to us: the medical profession no longer believed in the six-month "deadline," while the others used it to limit payment for treatment they deemed "useless for such a chronic condition." The withholding of professional therapy, specifically, to help Tracy became painfully apparent in the months and years to come.

On a summer afternoon, Bill and I received a crash course on finding a safe, clean, caring "rehabilitation and care center" for Tracy. There were insurance limitations as to what sort of rehabilitation and care facility Tracy could qualify for. Again, the OHSU staff made our quest so much easier: they understood rules, regulations, financial limits and eligibility requirements so we got a list of a few facilities to visit.

We drove over much of the Portland Metro area on the one afternoon we had to find Tracy a new "home" away from home. We learned at the first facility we visited that there was a short cut to determining whether a facility was one we thought would be good enough for Tracy: smell.

We visited three centers. The first two smelled absolutely awful. I'm sure keeping a facility like this smelling good takes effort. But, no one could have wanted to live in those two places. When we walked into the last facility, it smelled... not at all. It was lighter inside than the first two, and it seemed much newer. We had called ahead to all three facilities and this was the only one that had "time" to spare for us. A representative from the first facility we visited said that we shouldn't expect too much: after all, we were searching for a place for someone "on welfare." At the third institution, we were met by the administrative coordinator and the social worker, and we were allowed to talk with nursing and therapy staff. We saw some patient rooms, the dining room and therapy rooms. Based on a quick visit, it certainly seemed better than the others. It was located west of the Metro area which made it a little closer for Tracy's friends from Lincoln City to visit. And, we had run out of time. So, we asked them to be ready to receive Tracy when OHSU released him.

Up to the day Tracy moved to the rehabilitation and care center twenty miles west of where we lived, I was at the hospital or in Lincoln City taking care of things for Tracy every day except one. On the days I was in Lincoln City, I called the hospital for updates. On the days I was unable to visit, Alison went to see Tracy.

Sometimes Bill went to see Tracy, but not often. When he did go to the hospital, he spent most of the time in the waiting room or the coffee shop. He seemed to tune out when I told him the latest information about Tracy. I got the feeling that he didn't want to know the details because if he didn't know, then "it" wasn't so bad -- he wouldn't know how badly this stroke had hammered Tracy. Bill minimized my concerns and downplayed what I reported the medical team was saying. He would force a smile and respond with some variation of forceful enthusiasm at the end of his attention span: "Well, it sounds like good news! He's getting better and better and in no time, we'll have our life back!" Finally, I came to believe that he didn't want to hear anything but when this ordeal would be over, so I stopped telling him very much. We had shared everything for thirty-eight years and moved through our life together pretty much in tandem. So this was new territory, not really communicating any more. I no longer had the sounding board that I'd had since Bill and I had come together many years ago. I thought we were in for some rough times, but I had neither the strength nor the will to deal with it at this point. In fairness to Bill, he was there when I specifically asked him or when he thought that I needed him. He also usually did what I specifically asked of him, such as shave Tracy when he had grown substantial facial hair. That was a big deal because Tracy was on blood thinners and if he suffered a cut or scratch, he would bleed excessively. Bill never had shaved anyone other than himself. And also in fairness, Bill was still dealing with his own physical therapy for his knee. He didn't get his brace off until mid-July, six weeks after Tracy's stroke.

Later, I came to understand that some people hate going to the hospital to visit people they care about. Bill had served in Vietnam. I think hospitals forced him to face injury and death and he didn't like it. He hated being in hospitals. I didn't know it. His way of getting through a situation he couldn't control was either to make light of it or to craft a detailed military operations plan to defeat it: Nothing in between. Another person who couldn't stand to see Tracy not as he used to be was Alison's daughter, Tracy's niece Nicole. Nicole adored Tracy. She and her mother had lived with Tracy when she was little while her mother and Tracy were students at the University of Oregon. I remember walking into their kitchen one morning to find Tracy and four-year-old Nicole covered in flour. Nicole was "helping" Tracy make bread. The activity included throwing flour. Nicole to this day loves to cook and to garden. She got both interests from Tracy during the time they lived together in Eugene. Nicole never visited Tracy in any facility. She just couldn't. She tried once, but sat in the car in the parking lot for hours and then left. She beat herself up about it, but it was months later before she saw him after he had his stroke.

I believe that Bill looked upon the move from the hospital to the rehab center as a big step toward Tracy's independence and our "getting our life back." Bill believed it would mean that I would spend less time with Tracy and more with him. Life would be returning to normal. We were to discover that "normal" wasn't going to show up very soon.

Chapter 5:
Closing Down a House and
Closing Up a Studio...

For now, I felt a little as if I were running at top speed over cracking ice and the edge of the pond was very far away.

Since his medical issues were beyond my control or ability, my first priority was finding and protecting Tracy's paintings and photographs – and other projects I came to realize he was working on. I also needed to make decisions about his house and his possessions.

His friends had some specific ideas. Glass artist Kelly and former studio mate Jane wanted to leave everything precisely like it was so it would look the same to Tracy when he came home. One of them had read somewhere that it was important for people who left their home unexpectedly to return to find everything the same. We laughed when we decided that that didn't include leaving the refrigerator untouched or the garbage and recycling under the sink. Early on, none of us had a realistic concept of how long he would be "away." Even though his friends said they would come by everyday and keep a close watch on his house, I was uncomfortable with that solution. It asked a great deal of his friends, and I felt I was ultimately responsible for protecting the few material things that mattered to Tracy – but I lived one-hundred-plus miles away. We talked about the best course of action over the next few days.

Tracy's friends have been his friends for many years. They come from different walks of life and each loves Tracy for himself and for what he has brought to their community. I don't know all the details of how and when Tracy met these friends, but I experienced their selflessness and commitment to getting Tracy back. They knew the "current" Tracy better than I did: he'd been living at the Coast in their community for ten years.

I think the first time I met Jane was when she and Tracy were sharing studio space. She's a gifted photographer who finds and releases the secrets that an image offers. Jane had been a neighbor of Tracy's. She and her husband, Scott, live in Taft, a older, tiny community within Lincoln City that is home to many artists. It was at Jane's and Scott's house one very cold and rainy July 4th that Bill and I first met Sharon. Sharon was bundled up cooking chicken wings on the BBQ. We chatted a bit and she said she recently had moved to Lincoln City. As the afternoon unfolded, we tasted some of those chicken wings and Bill went back and told her, "You know, those are pretty darned good!" He said to me, "Boy, she has some cooking talent; she oughta be a chef." When he said that to someone else at the party, they laughed and said, "She is. She's the new chef at the Lincoln City Culinary Center." Sharon is a "take charge" person. She lets people wander around a subject for not very long before she takes the subject by the horns and "does something." One of the many concrete and supremely practical ways Sharon helped me was letting me stay at her house while I was working at Tracy's. It allowed me to rest. I discovered that when I "slept" at Tracy's, I didn't sleep. I got up and worked. Jane, Sharon and Tracy shared an interest in spending time and energy at the local Highway 101 Gym, which is run by Silkie. I first met Silkie in the OHSU Neurosciences ICU waiting room. I discovered then she was the person who first saw Tracy a few hours after his stroke and called the ambulance. I will always be grateful for her keen power of observation and good judgment. Tracy worked out with Richard, a body builder. Jane struggles with massive health issues and used the gym to get the most she could out of her frail body. Whenever she helped me for Tracy, and she helped so much in a number of ways, I always marveled at her sweet smile.

Kelly, oh Kelly. How do I begin to describe one of the greatest loves of my brother's life? A truly gifted artist, who blows glass into the most astounding and breathtakingly beautiful shapes and colors, Kelly has personal layers and textures that make her as interesting a human being as she is an artist. Multi-faceted with many interests and talents, Kelly's gentle heart and poetic soul wander the earth seeking goodness amongst many lesser and more mortal beings. Like many who are good at what they do, she has had her share of "relationship" messes. Kelly and Tracy can – and have – spent hours talking animatedly about an infinite number of subjects, solving no problems but having a whale of a good time in each other's company. I think Tracy was impressed with Kelly's artistic ability, saw much untapped potential for her to expand and share her gifts, and loved the sensitive, vulnerable but strong being he glimpsed underpinning her surface. He told me more than once she has no idea how good of an artist she really is. Tracy never married. He said it was because he chose to live as a starving artist and wouldn't foist that life off on anyone, much less someone he loved. He felt he had insufficient resources -- not nothing, but insufficient -- to offer anyone he loved. He offered Kelly what he had: a great appreciation of her art, love of her caring heart and mentoring where he felt he could offer something helpful. As artists and philosophers waxing poetic over great coffees at Pacific Grind on rainy afternoons, they are two peas in a pod. After Tracy's "incident," Kelly told me she was rudderless and adrift without Tracy. The hole his absence left in his community was immense.

Matt and Tracy knew each other from years ago at a local gallery, where Matt worked and Tracy showed his art. They also were neighbors, and often Matt and sometimes his wife, Tracy, would take walks with Tracy around the lovely Siletz Bay area of the little town of Taft. We laughed over the years as we talked about Tracy: "Your" Tracy or "My" Tracy? Matt and Tracy have been married since they were young and are the parents of a splendid son, industrious Harry, who helped me find Tracy's computer secrets and set up "Support for Tracy" on Facebook. Matt and his wife love this particular area of the Coast, and they were very creative about work: they cobbled together jobs so they could live there and raise their son in a small, friendly, beautiful community on the Oregon Coast. As far as I knew, Matt's Tracy had substituted and then taught at the local school and worked seasonally at Volta Glass Gallery, along with "my" Tracy. When "my" Tracy had his stroke, Matt's Tracy stepped in fulltime at the Glass Gallery. She's a "glue person," someone who brings people and things together in a happy way. Matt's Tracy has a great laugh. She just makes people around her feel good. Matt and "his" Tracy also are active in Theatre West as actors, directors, stagehands – doing anything and everything that the small local theatre requires. "My" Tracy told me once that he suffered from a complicated relationship with his actor friends when they were on stage at Theatre West. He always went to performances because he wanted to support his friends, but he was terrified that in the confines of that little but very live space, they might flub a line and he would be so worried for them. He found that he fretted over such an inevitable occurrence much more intently than they did. Matt and Tracy and their son, Harry, were frequent and quiet visitors who came to be with Tracy at each stage of his recovery.

I'm not sure where "my" Tracy met Robin, but she's good friends with Matt and "his" Tracy, and is also a school teacher who gives a big part of her heart to Theatre West and to her own photography and writing. One of the funniest portrayals I ever saw was Robin in her role in *NunSense* for Theatre West. She and "my" Tracy also were neighbors for awhile in a great older apartment building that overlooked the ocean – and took the brunt of the wind as well. From that apartment, I believe she moved into her first house as a homeowner – the one where she offered space for Tracy's things in the garage. I think some outdoor chairs made it to her deck, as well.

Whenever Bill and I visited Tracy in earlier days, I pushed to visit Barking Dog Organic Farm, south of town, just east of Highway 101 up the Siletz Highway. In such a gorgeous setting, Dave and Heidi grow perfect veggies and shelter various rescue animals. Tracy routinely went to see what else they had at their store because Dave was very good at getting the first and the best of something from the farmers' co-op. Heidi uses their barn for other things since she's a sculptor. A tiny person, she crafts intricate tiny moving sculptures or huge metal art pieces. One year, she made several small metal dolls with moving arms and legs from the parts of old manual typewriters. Trust me, they were delightfully creative. One huge piece is *Sparky The Dragon*, about ten feet tall and now on display at Lincoln City's Regatta Park.

Ultimately, Tracy's landlord, Chris, made the decision for us. Kelly had made sure that Tracy's rent was paid for July, but unbeknownst to any of us, Chris and Tracy had had preliminary discussions about Tracy moving because Chris's mother wanted to move into the little house. She had lived in it with her husband many years ago and now, suffering with early onset Alzheimer's, she wanted to return to a place with happy memories. One day when I was in Lincoln City at Tracy's house, Chris and his family were visiting from their home in Texas. He came by with his family and we talked. He was so gracious, and we decided an August move would suit both of us.

Now we had a direction. We needed to find a place for Tracy's things. In the last year or so, Robin had moved into her first house. It had a two-car garage that she never used. I asked her why, since everyone knows it rains a lot at the Coast, and I thought it would be a lot more comfortable for her to get in-and-out of her car in a dry garage. She laughed and said she was used to the rain and besides, she never figured out how to open the garage door from the outside! She offered her garage for us to store Tracy's things from his kitchen, bedroom and living room, his camping gear, and all the odd-shaped items -- like the old giant lighting system living in the refrigerator in the garage at Tracy's house. We could add two of his large worktables and still be able to put Luna, his 4-Runner, in the garage, too.

During my many trips back-and-forth that summer, I kept myself entertained by keeping track of how long each trip took, and counting the number of passing lanes on Highway 18. I preferred the route using Highway 99W to I-5 which I find to be boring. Highway 99 goes through more hills and valleys and offers splendid views of sky, fields and vineyards. The 120-mile trip usually took me just over two hours, one-way. I avoided travel on Fridays and Sundays during nice weather because that's when everyone headed to-and-from the Coast. When it gets very hot in the Willamette Valley, which is where the Portland area nestles to the north, everyone tries to get to the beach because it's foggy and cool. The heat in the Valley pulls the clouds and fog in from the ocean over the first mile or so of the Coast like a big, cool fuzzy blanket. There are a few little towns drivers slow down to get through, like Dundee. Dundee is a darling little town in the middle of Wine Country, and Highway 99W goes right through the middle of it. Drivers call it the "Dundee Crawl." The whole route makes its way from suburbs, through rolling hills spotted with Oregon oak and vineyards, to the eastern edge of the Coast range. From there, the hills get higher and are covered with evergreen trees – where they haven't been clear-cut. The last segment of the trip is along the Salmon River which sparkles in sunshine and provides damp edges for ferns and skunk cabbage.

On one of my first trips to Tracy's house, I tried to figure out things like where and how he paid for lights, heat, internet/TV/phone. I went through his desk and the suspicious absence of paperwork led me to believe he conducted most of these transactions online. Where to start? I thought of Harry, son of Matt and "his" Tracy. Harry was about 12-years-old when he and "my" Tracy first became acquainted. "My" Tracy helped him create his first website. Now a high-school senior, I just knew that Harry was the man for the job. I emailed him, told him my predicament, and asked if he thought he could help. He was wonderful. Over the next several months, he led me through the world of banking and finance online: how to find and decipher online bills that had no paper copies; how to get Tracy's passwords so I could enter his accounts (that's still a secret); how to keep Tracy's small website business going (Harry took it over and ran it, but we had big arguments about payment ... He wouldn't accept any payments for his outstanding work. I convinced him to keep what he needed to pay necessary bills to keep the business afloat.) And, he instructed me in the mysterious "i-world" of iMacs, iPhones, iPods and iPads.

Wonderful Harry came by before and after work to help me figure out things with the computer. Harry said it wasn't a problem: one could get only so excited about folding shirts for Old Navy. That was his summer job before he left for college. Harry began boxing up Tracy's computers. I was concerned about leaving them in the now-unoccupied house. Just to be doubly safe, I bought another hard drive for storage at Harry's suggestion and he backed up everything on Tracy's computers. He said no doubt it was redundancy because he knew Tracy backed up everything, but we wanted to be positive that everything was safe. Over the next few weeks, as I visited Tracy's house, I found more computer "stuff," like a box of stray cords in the attic. I wasn't sure how any of it might relate to the setup in his office. I decided the things related to computers in his office must be current. The other stuff was ... extra? not working? old? At his desk, I found a writing pad on which he had jotted down some notes, including what looked like a case number, something about having contacted Apple about a problem with his computer. Harry and I (mostly Harry) pieced it together, and I called Apple. It seemed Tracy already had contacted them and they were waiting for him to bring it in so they could look at it and fix it. I made arrangements to take his errant computer to Apple. As I looked further around his desk, I discovered a very impressive metal contraption underneath it that was labeled "Monster." Well that made my day. He was keeping a "Monster" under his desk. I thought of Harry Potter and the textbook he got to study Monsters ... the one that, when opened, chased Harry about his bedroom trying to eat his feet. I made sure the "Monster" under Tracy's desk didn't have any way to open and snap at my feet! Spending time alone in the house of a loved one can make you a bit loopy.

Harry's dad, Matt, came by and took apart Tracy's TV cable system so I could return the box and wires and stop the service to Tracy's house since no one was watching TV there. At Charter Communications, we decided to leave the internet service on so we could use the computer. They said they had paperless billing with Tracy and the bill was automatically paid from his credit union account, but they also said there was a past due amount. I paid it and returned the equipment. I wanted to be sure his account was O.K. for the future when he would need it. Matt also hooked me up with Tracy's landlord for his storefront studio. The rent was already due for the next month and I didn't know what arrangements had been made for first and last month's rent. I paid the rent due and gave notice.

Tracy had some great houseplants including two indoor trees. Kelly took one of them to Volta Glass Gallery, where Tracy had worked and Kelly showed her glass artwork. The others we checked and watered. Over the next few weeks, his plants went to new homes with old friends. Kelly kept bringing in the mail until I notified the post office and changed Tracy's address to ours in Beaverton.

As I looked around Tracy's house, in essence, peering into each corner of his life, I marveled at the life he had made for himself. Several partly completed projects were apparent: photographs, posters, a book being crafted, paintings in all stages of creation, including some requiring maintenance and repair, journals filled with ideas for paintings and artwork for a CD jacket. This was the part of Tracy's life I hadn't seen in detail because it was born after he moved to the Coast. Before then, he'd completed his masters in fine arts (MFA) in visual design with an emphasis in photography. An MFA is what's called a "terminal" degree – it's the highest degree there is in fine arts, and it's equivalent to a Ph.D. in other disciplines.

Over fourteen years, Tracy dedicated himself to trying to teach photography at the college level, using his experience and education. He wanted to teach, and he was good at it. He taught at three different Oregon universities, in all three cases as either an adjunct professor or in a temporary professional position. He taught photo I and II, large format and a senior seminar in advanced photography at the University of Oregon. At Willamette University, he taught photography, including a class on multi-media production and manipulative photography. After that year, unbeknownst to him until later, most of his Willamette students requested to talk with the hiring committee to tell them what it was like to be in his class – and that they should hire him. Tracy was a visiting artist at the local community college as well.

He, and the rest of his family and friends, assumed in all three situations that successful completion of a year in a temporary position likely would lead to a full-time permanent college-level teaching position. He completed each contract and received very strong evaluations. He applied for permanent, full-time teaching positions in photography at all three universities. He also applied to the University of Montana for a photography teaching position. He was not hired at any of the four schools in any position, much less as a photography instructor in a permanent, full-time college-level position. At all three Oregon universities, women were hired to fill vacant positions, including one who had been one of Tracy's former students. He does not know who was hired at the University of Montana. As I've gotten older, I've wondered if the playing field is ever level. I'd lived the limitations of a woman trying to advance on a professional employment track, finding I spent more time in "interim" and "temporary" positions than winning "real" titles with commensurate pay. Finally, companies and institutions, including universities, had begun to get serious about hiring women in professional positions. There was a great deal of lost time to make up. The field tilted again, and Tracy wasn't on the winning end.

In my opinion, it's easier to land a job with a master's in business administration than it is to find work with a master's in fine arts. Artists are different kinds of animals. They follow their own star. And, they often pay the price for being outside the norm. I have women friends who fought fiercely to land tenured-track positions in academia. They understood they had to be willing to go to places no one else wanted to be in order to climb onto the starting rung. As I contemplate what I know of their lives, the ones who needed the out-of-doors as Tracy does, struggled more than those who could make their art inside a building. One of my friends isn't living her life; she's making do, having made major compromises on where she lives and works, marking time – now for more than 25 years.

Tracy found himself staring at student loans with no way to repay them if he couldn't find a professional-level job in his field. I don't know of other positions he pursued or other jobs he sought. After the fourth rejection, he decided he'd try being an artist instead of teaching about it. And, he'd expand his horizons to include paint on canvas. Thus, he moved to the Oregon Coast and began a new life. I saw the results as I looked around his house. This artist was, indeed, productive.

I put out the word that I needed boxes to pack Tracy's things. Every time I returned to Lincoln City, I found more boxes stacked in the living room. Later I discovered that was mostly Heidi's doing. I started looking in every box Tracy had stored upstairs, under the stairs, in the pantry, in his office, out in the garage and its back room. Most of the boxes were full, but I checked to be sure there was no unused space. Later when he began going through his boxes, I thought he'd start laughing about how I filled them. He organized by similar items. I organized by size, shape, and weight. I've always been a big fan of using sheets, towels and sweatshirts to balance out otherwise heavy boxes filled with breakable or heavy items. I opened yet another box of journals and books and nestled inside the box was an Indian brass bowl. Inside the bowl was a small slip of paper. In Tracy's unique lettering was the word "Simplify." It was a nice day so the windows were open. I'm glad the next door neighbors weren't there. I howled with laughter. Over the next six weeks, I went up-and-down those steep, narrow stairs so many times, dragging boxes and equipment downstairs, carrying paintings and boxes in-and-out of the garage, packing up the pantry and distributing food to friends, stripping his bed and taking comforters home to be cleaned. Tracy still used "college furniture" for shelving: concrete blocks and boards. Gosh, those are heavy to move around!

Every closet was full of "something." In one closet I found lots of DVDs. Out in the garage on a shelf I found lots of videos. Harry and I packed them all. In a little nook under the eaves I found his computer boxes and an amazing array of cords. I put them in a box, dragged them downstairs, and gave them to Wonderful Harry to sort out. I found Tracy's wetsuit. It went with his kayak that was parked out in back of his house. He lived in an ideal place: he had only to get the kayak across his little neighborhood street and he could launch it into the creek that flowed into the river, that went to the bay, that went to the ocean. One time he called me from his kayak in the middle of Siletz Bay to tell me that the seals had surrounded him and were looking at him with big brown eyes.

Each time I returned home, I'd pack the car with things I thought Tracy would want to see. Somehow I recognized that it would be a long time before he returned "home," and that part of that sojourn would be living at our house. I wished to put things there that I thought mattered a lot to him to make it feel more like home. I brought various items: some early journals he'd written, as well as his beloved espresso maker. I dismissed any thought that he would not be making the return journey.

Packing up his kitchen was unexpectedly hard for me. Maybe it was our shared love of good food served well. Maybe it was that we had traveled to many places where food was appreciated and we enjoyed the heck out of this together. Tracy meticulously had collected bright-colored dishes and bowls through the years. He had selected his glasses and coffee cups so they felt good held in your hand. I could so clearly see him bringing a mug of coffee to Bill, lovingly made with his espresso machine and decorated on top with foam, who would take a big sip, close his eyes, smile, and say, "Ah, the Elixir of the Gods!" And it was. I have never had coffee as good as Tracy's. His pantry included all sorts of nuts and seeds – I kept finding packets of flax seeds! – and I marveled at his branching out into Asian and Indian and fusion cuisine. My preferred tastes are pretty much Italian, French and American with maybe a bit of Spanish tossed in. Obviously, Tracy had gone exploring farther afield. I packed up the herbs, spices, and seeds that looked like they would stand the test of time and gave away much of the rest. Jane and I together individually wrapped his dishes and glasses and cups. Jane asked if it would be O.K. to wrap a stack of dishes together. I asked instead that they be wrapped individually. Somehow, I felt that if we took the best care we could with his things, neither he nor his things would be broken. Keeping his things safe might translate to his being safe. As I wrapped and packed each item, they were so strongly reminiscent of Tracy. It was a comfort to be that close to him, and a challenge not to burst into tears at the same time when I thought of why I was doing this.

Rather than waste time going out to eat, or trying to fix food at his house at the same time I was concentrating on closing down the house, I became a big fan of Builder Bars: lots of protein. In the course of those six weeks, I lost 28 pounds. That was a loss I could afford. I was building a pattern of my visits: spending the days at Tracy's house or on his business and then meeting his various friends for dinner. Mostly we met at a great local restaurant, La Roca, where we caught up with each other and listened to whoever had seen Tracy most recently. I thanked them for taking me in, because after all, I didn't live there and Tracy was *their* friend, not me. I was greeted by a loud "That's not true, you are OUR friend now." And they proved it, again and again.

Because I didn't yet have Power of Attorney, I was unable to get enough information to see to whom the money that was automatically coming out of Tracy's credit union accounts was going. While individual representatives of the various utility, communication or credit card companies were sorry about his troubles, officially they couldn't talk with me -- until I could provide them with a Power of Attorney document. I sent several letters, explaining what happened and that I was in the process of getting the Power of Attorney and asked them to at least highlight his account, not accept any charges and not charge him interest for something he couldn't help. That bought me a little time, but I moved expeditiously to figure out what to do so that costs would not mount further. I thought I'd put my finger in the dike to prevent any further expenditures. I was wrong. Each time I checked, more money was going out of his account and onto his credit cards even though I had asked specifically that no more money flow from his account. There were automatic and pre-authorized payments that I was powerless to stop. His account balance bottomed out. Tracy owned a savings account and a checking account plus two credit cards – one for business and one for personal use – with the credit union. He had used the business card as a backup to the checking account: if the checking account went below $5, a cash loan was taken from his credit card at a high interest rate. In addition, each credit-card bill came with a minimum monthly payment. I couldn't get the credit union to stop these transactions until I could complete the Power of Attorney.

I thought I had the problem solved after I provided the credit union copies of the Power of Attorney. Apparently not. As soon as I had access to his accounts, I could see that banking activity continued: money was going out to pay bills on automatic pilot. I was one step behind, trying to fathom which bills were still coming in and being paid even though I had asked that everything just stop until I could get a handle on the situation. I tracked down all the external bills and got the companies (communications, phone and utilities, for example) to suspend the automatic billing and send me paper bills. I gave each of them copies of the Power of Attorney. I paid final bills in full because I wanted good credit for him later. It took me two cycles to get them to stop paying the rent. But his landlord, Chris, was great, returning the last check and accepting my word that Tracy had paid first and last month's rent. This was complicated because while I found a copy of the rental agreement, I couldn't find a copy of the original check that had paid first and last when Tracy first rented his house. In turn, the landlord's mother had no record either.

The biggest problem was the credit union. No money from outside was going into either the savings or the checking account. I had stopped all the other bills. The few automatic bills now coming in were from the credit union itself: the two credit cards and their monthly minimum balance payments. The credit union was automatically transferring a cash loan/advance from Tracy's business account credit card to pay the minimum payments due on their own credit cards. The savings account went down to almost zero and every time money "automatically" transferred from savings to checking, there was a $5 fee. There were seemingly endless transfers that I kept trying to get stopped. The whole business reminded me of the Disney movie version of the "Sorcerer's Apprentice," when Mickey Mouse was overcome by buckets and brooms and water. The water just kept coming! I asked that they freeze his accounts and suspend interest and penalty charges on the credit cards since there was a clear medical reason they were not being paid. While other creditors worked with me, the credit union did not. They continued to charge interest and fees, going from an amount due of about $9,500 to more than $17,000 by the time they sent the "bill" to collections. Subsequently, I worked with their collection agency, which determined, after a year, that the bill was uncollectible. I was in regular contact with the collection agency during that time, and it did not charge additional interest or fees. As I slogged my way through this mess, I wondered how people who had a stroke, like Tracy, could ever fix something like the credit union's actions on their own.

All these trips were building toward a crescendo: Moving Day. I enlisted family and friends to help. In the Saturday convoy from Beaverton were Bill, Alison and my son, Mitch, driving their respective pickup trucks. Good-hearted Tim, a friend of Alison's, rode with Mitch. He and Mitch did much of the heavy lifting in the next couple of days. My friend Mary brought her Subaru down on Sunday morning because we had measured it earlier and found two of Tracy's favorite, big, but not sturdily framed paintings fit perfectly into the back of her car.

We gutted Tracy's house. His things were placed in four places: a climatized storage unit for his work materials and paintings for sale; Robin's garage for his household goods, big, weirdly shaped items, and Luna, his 4-Runner SUV; a second storage unit for art not for sale; and our house for things we wanted closer to Tracy when he was ready for them. Matt and Jane and Faith came by before or after work to help pack. Kelly came over and took charge of packing all the glass. We called it her Glass Protection Program. And it worked: we lost no blown glass. Tracy had several pieces of her work there because he was photographing it for a book.

I asked Matt to go by Lincoln City Storage and check out two different units: a 10-foot x10-foot and a 20-foot x10-foot to see which he thought we should rent. He thought the larger one would make sense because it would offer the freedom for people moving paintings around in it if someone wanted to see them. He also suggested which side of the facility to use: the one out of the wind and driving rain so when the door was open, the insides would be more protected. I never would have thought of that until it was too late. We got two sets of keys. One stayed with Matt.

The plan on Saturday was to finish staging and move the paintings and photographs going to the second storage unit, almost all in Jane and Scott's covered trailer. Once the Beaverton contingent arrived later on Saturday, we'd use those pickups and that muscle to move the heavier stuff and as many of the things going to Robin's as we could that day. Jane and Scott had finished moving the paintings to the second storage unit, and we were waiting for the group to arrive from Beaverton.

Sharon stood up, looked around, and said, "What are we waiting for? Let's see how much we can get done before they get here!" She called Doug – another staunch friend with a big pickup. She called Silkie and Richard, the Body Builder, both from Highway 101 Gym. Scott returned with an empty trailer thinking his work was done. Poor man. Scott, Richard and Doug manhandled Tracy's 225-pound printer around sharp corners and down the steep, narrow stairs out to Doug's pickup. That along with a heavy, long, black cupboard to store boxes of photographs, a stand-up light and more boxes travelled to the storage unit.

Boxes of books and paper and paintings available for sale were loaded into the trailer along with cans of paint, boxes of tints, mineral spirits, alcohol, palette knives and paint brushes. Scott ended up working like a mad man, stacking all the boxes at the back end of the storage unit, floor to ceiling. In went two printers, the big one covered by an old bright purple (Tracy's alma mater, University of Washington, Husky color!) down sleeping bag. They came back for more. Tracy's red couch, a gift from another friend, Anita, in years past, was loaded into the pickup and taken to the storage unit. We laughed about people sitting on it while viewing paintings in the storage unit. Old stereo speakers went in along with a few boxes of nonperishable food. Big, funny-shaped items went into the storage unit: a large, heavy, fragile vase that looked like an Indian drum, a giant easel, a TV, a room-sized rolled-up braided rug, stretcher boards, gessoed canvas (canvas with a plaster of paris and glue preparation), rolled linen and some sort of professional speaker system that had hung out at Tracy's for years. We were on a roll. We emptied the living room and a good part of the garage's back room.

When the Beaverton group arrived, everyone paused to meet each other and then went right to work. By the time we all dragged into La Roca for dinner on Saturday night, the house was pretty much empty. We had loaded the trucks with things for our house and for Robin's and left them tucked in next to the garage overnight. We put his bed in the garage, too. The Coast is rainy. In the morning, we went back and finished packing what needed to go into the garage. Tracy's pink "viewing chair" sat above the fray on a worktable. At the very end, Mitch backed Luna into the garage. Bill stayed another day, but the rest of the family and my friend, Mary, their vehicles fully loaded, went back on Sunday. Robin, Faith, and I cleaned the silent house. Matt took the garbage to the dump and any remaining boxes to recycling.

Tracy had carried many things around for years. When people don't have much, they happily accept gifts and hand-me-downs and then keep them just in case. We took everything the next step to protect them until he could reclaim his life. It wasn't up to us to decide what he should keep. In the months to come, some of his things went to other, temporary, homes. Sharon, for example, needed a kitchen table and chairs and a bed for guests and his TV was bigger than hers, so they went to her house. It seemed better to let his things be useful for his friends.

I took one last walk around Tracy's house, made sure I had the house key, locked everything and went across the street to Gary's house. Through the years Gary had built shipping boxes and other specialized things for Tracy. He also was one of the many people who went clear to Portland to visit Tracy while he was in the hospital. Gary was a friend of the landlord, Chris. By previous arrangement, I handed the key to Gary and said we were finished. Just as I left, a little lady on a bicycle with a flag on it stopped me. She said her name was Maggie. She wanted to thank me for the Support for Tracy Facebook page because, she said, she was just a neighbor who was concerned about Tracy, and it was a superb means of tracking what was happening with him. I thanked her for her good thoughts for Tracy and said I couldn't take credit for the Facebook page. I told her it was mostly Harry. She said she knew him. And so I left Tracy's house and neighborhood. His things were spread all over now, but maybe they'd be an even stronger anchor that way, pulling him back home when it was time.

Chapter 6:
The Hows and Whys
of Rehabilitation Centers ...

In mid-July, I had gone to Lincoln City to do more packing because we didn't know the exact date or time of Tracy's move from OHSU's Acute Care Unit to the rehabilitation center and because things needed to be taken care of back in Tracy's hometown. In the mysterious ways of medical transfers, we heard nothing for days, and then, when I was in Lincoln City, we were told that Tracy was being moved *that day* to the rehab center. For a long time, I harbored resentment about the way Bill handled the move into the rehab center. I also have not forgiven myself for not being there to take care of the move the way I wanted it done. I wanted Bill to do it *my* way. He couldn't see what the big deal was. An ambulance transported Tracy. Bill worked hard to move all the "stuff" that had accumulated in Tracy's hospital room over the twenty-six days he'd been at OHSU -- plants, banners, pictures, cards, a painting, clothes -- out to his new room at the rehabilitation center. The place was run by professionals, after all, and Bill assumed they knew what they were doing. He made sure Tracy was in his room, and then he left. He had made dinner reservations for us because I was driving back from Lincoln City, Tracy had moved toward independence, and because he wanted us to celebrate "getting our life back." I wasn't quite sure how that was happening, but was too tired to argue.

On the last morning Tracy was at OHSU, Bill reported to friends in an email that Tracy looked and acted better than he'd seen him since he had the stroke. He said his eyes were open much of the time; he laughed and spoke, and he got his own water bottle from the bedside table and drank from it. Bill wrote friends about the facility Tracy was moving to and said they already had gone online and looked at Tracy's website and were duly impressed. I guessed he thought that must mean they understood they were getting an important patient? While Tracy's blood pressure remained high, Bill took what he saw as good news.

On the first morning Tracy was at the rehabilitation center, Bill sent another email.

"Hi All -- Tracy had a rough night after I left the nursing home. He ate a big dinner and then got up to sit in a chair. His blood pressure did a number on him, and he got dizzy and fell. And then he fell again trying to get back to bed, scraping his side a bit when he banged into the air conditioner. He then threw up his dinner. Wendy was with him this morning, and he still was having trouble keeping food down. She got some cottage cheese, and he was eating tiny bites and keeping it down, at least for now. The big problem continues to be his blood pressure. They still haven't found the combination, so it goes up and down, causing trouble both ways. His mind mostly is alert, and yesterday he seemed more like the Tracy I know. But Wendy said this morning that he was not as alert and talkative. So, two steps forward and one back. Let's hope the steps forward continue at a good pace. As far as nursing homes go, this one seems decent, and I think when Tracy settles into a routine things will improve. Here's hoping, anyway. Cheers, bill"

When Alison and I arrived at the rehabilitation center about 9 a.m., Tracy was in bed and the lights were out in his room. I opened the door and turned on the bathroom light with the door partly shut so the light wouldn't be so bright. He groaned. I asked him what was wrong … why wasn't he up and dressed? Had he eaten? He said he wasn't feeling well. At the hospital, he wasn't invited to get up. They got him up. Here, it appeared to be more "if you feel like it." When he turned over, he winced. Again, I asked what was wrong. He said he'd fallen the night before and he pointed at the air conditioner unit he'd hit. I examined his side and found it scraped and scabbed over with a very big bruise. No one had cleaned it or treated it.

First, I was furious with Bill. Somehow (irrationally, I know), I concluded that if he had made more of a fuss when Tracy was admitted the day before instead of trying to get out of there as soon as possible, they wouldn't have left him alone, and neither his falling last night nor his still being in bed this morning would have happened. And I just knew that if I'd been there instead, somehow I would have prevented this very poor start at this "care" facility. After fuming for a few minutes, I walked over to the nurses' station and asked to see his chart. We had a discussion about what I expected of them and that included, at a minimum, safety and getting him up for breakfast. I also waited for someone to examine and treat his injury. They said breakfast was over but they could maybe get him a tray. I agreed that would be a very good idea, and asked specifically for cottage cheese. Not because he likes it; he doesn't. But I was looking for something with protein that would calm his stomach.

Since they didn't respond as fast as I wanted them to (as in, immediately – I know, another example of my irrationality), I went in search of the kitchen and wandered into the "other" wing of the care facility. That opened my eyes. Many rehabilitation and care facilities have two wings: the one with people who might get better and the one for people who don't. At that time, if a patient didn't perform adequately, didn't show "continued improvement," they were wheeled down to the fork in the hallway and melded into the group of almost motionless and mostly silent human beings sitting or slumping in the hallway waiting for something, anything, nothing.

Beside all the other challenges Tracy had with eating, some of the medication he was given triggered heartburn, so he was even less interested in food. By the time he came to the rehabilitation center, he had lost almost 40 pounds, and he wasn't that heavy to begin with.

We got him changed, face washed, hair combed, teeth brushed, a little food in him, and he was exhausted. He'd had a big couple of days, so we said we would be back the next day. When I went again to the nurses' station, I asked for an appointment with the head nurse on Monday morning. When I checked in that night with the nurse overseeing Tracy's room, I was told he was having a good night and that there would be no more problems with his falling out of bed.

I returned to the rehabilitation center the next morning. I discovered why there had been no problems with Tracy falling out of bed: they had tied him in. I told them he was not to be tied in bed. There was a rail he could use. They said they didn't trust him not to leave his bed without a staff person present. I asked if they had asked him not to. They said they just assumed he wouldn't understand or wouldn't obey. We had further discussion. Tracy agreed he would not get out of bed unless staff was present, and he would use the call button to get staff to come to him. They agreed not to tie him in bed. Then we got on with breakfast and clean up. He again asked that the lights be kept off and the curtains drawn. Light in general made him cringe. He asked that the door to his room be kept shut because it was so noisy outside his room. I didn't think it was *that* bad, but it obviously bothered him a great deal. He also was agitated by the smell of Pinesol used to clean the floors. I asked the staff not to clean the floor in his room unless he was not there. To this day, he cannot stand the smell of Pinesol. It appeared that he was becoming even more sensitive to everything: light, sound, smells, and tastes all elicited strong and negative reactions from him. Some of his complaints about smells were inaccurate: he complained about the smell of Clorox and there was no Clorox. He hated the Pinesol, but this "other" smell was also awful. We couldn't figure out what it was. Foods he had enjoyed before his stroke he no longer liked. Eggs were off the list, as was milk, other dairy products and hot peppers. But on the list was sugar. He'd never much liked sugar or processed foods, but now he couldn't get enough. Blood tests showed an elevated blood-sugar level.

When Alison came to visit later that day, she brought an electric toothbrush, a bigger comb easier for him to hold, and attachments to his razor so we could trim nose and ear hair he seemed to be growing. She also brought new socks, underwear, T-shirts and sweats because all his clothes were in Lincoln City and he hadn't needed much clothing at the hospital.

Tracy stayed at the rehabilitation center for seventy days. Again, except when in Lincoln City and one day in August, I saw Tracy every day. I counted the number of traffic signals between our house and the Center: twenty-six. I called every night to talk with the night nurse. I was either driving them crazy or assuring them that a whole bunch of people cared a great deal for Tracy and he was not a forgotten soul. We were all watching. Alison and I split shifts now: I went during the day; she went in the early evening. Often her brother, Mitch, would go after work. And Tracy's friends kept coming, too.

In the first few days he was at the rehabilitation center, Tracy, Alison, Bill and I met with staff to let them know what we expected for Tracy over the next several weeks: Get him ready to succeed at "rehab boot camp" in Portland. I asked for the meeting to nail down exactly how to proceed. I feared having one day blend into another with nothing specific happening. We all agreed on a plan that included daily therapy with the old "Triumvirate of Therapies" (physical, occupational and speech). Alison agreed to take the lead with the speech therapist and I asked Bill to do the same for physical therapy. I thought if they learned how to work with him in these areas, we could continue to help him when he no longer lived in a residential-care facility. We asked that close observation be made as to his reaction to the many, many pills he was taking. At that point, he was taking 12 medications several times a day, plus the medical staff was trying all sorts of things to get his nausea under control – strong anti-nausea pills before meals or, at one point, a Scopolomine patch. Too bad he wasn't getting the ocean cruise to go along with it! Our hope was to reduce the number of medications he was taking over time because almost all of them apparently caused troubling side effects.

We wanted him to become stronger, hence he must eat well and avoid vomiting. With the help of Tracy's friend, Jane, we introduced nutritious fresh fruit smoothies that they allowed us to make in his room. However, the rehabilitation center refused responsibility for making them or storing the raw materials to make them. I could understand that. Since I knew what was going into the smoothies, that was fine with me. (Although Nicole, Tracy's grand-niece, couldn't bring herself to come and see him, she loaned him her small refrigerator and we installed it in Tracy's room.) Tracy was at the beginning of a long road and we were asking him to perform at least as well as Hercules would under the circumstances. My family knew how I was when I got the bit between my teeth. They just let me run with it.

For the first time, while we were in a meeting with the rehabilitation center staff, it hit me: Tracy, eventually, was going to have to live at *our* house. Where else would he go? After all the treatment and rehabilitation and stabilizing, he would need to live somewhere besides a hospital or "facility." I looked at him at the meeting as we all sat around the table and saw no immediate possibility of his living independently. While I kept up my spirits by telling myself how well he was doing, I was also able to be pretty realistic about his actual progress toward recovery.

It's not hard to make a decision when there's nothing to decide. That's how I felt about what I needed to do for Tracy. The course of action was obvious to me. Questions and other choices didn't enter into the equation. Who we are today comes from where we've been. Past really is prologue.

Growing up, my immediate family was tight-knit. We depended upon ourselves and each other and no one else. And we were happy that way. The assault on that solid unit began with a scream early one bright April day when I was eight-years-old. I was outside, up a tree, watching morning unfold. I ran back to the house. Both my parents were in our bedroom, holding on to my almost six-year-old sister who was shrieking. Sherry never shrieked. Thus began a sad, frantic, terrifying, long journey that resulted more than two-years later in Sherry's death, my father's life-long struggle with alcohol, and the fracturing of my family. It was her death that broke us. We withstood the suffering and the fear and the anguish, even the bankruptcy, but our family couldn't survive her death. And yet, two years later my parents gave me the most marvelous gift: a baby brother. This was no easy task on their part. I remember being called to the school front office for a phone call one Tuesday morning in early October. Everybody knew why. My dad was calling to tell me I had a new brother or sister. I picked up the phone; everyone in the office was quiet and looking at me. I asked my dad if it was a boy or girl. He said, "Well, it has two ears, one on each side of its head." He followed with, "You have a baby brother named John Tracy." Tracy was my gift from my parents. I always looked after him. There was no decision to be made about it – he was coming home to Beaverton.

Because we truly didn't understand it, all of us glossed over a continuing giant impediment standing in Tracy's way: fatigue. We came to understand – Tracy showed us – how pervasive and insidious fatigue is for stroke victims. Just getting up in the morning and sitting on the side of the bed required immense concentration and strength. Sometimes even that was just too much. The combination of fatigue and dizziness that brought on nausea was pretty constant. Tracy mostly tried to beat them, work through them, find tools to accommodate them. But sometimes, he just had to stay still.

Alison and I discovered some holes in the daily fabric as we got used to the routine at the rehabilitation center. Because of his dizziness and his promise not to get up without help, Tracy had to wait for staff to have time for him in the mornings. Mornings are a very busy time in care facilities. I started getting there earlier in the morning to help him start his day because there were too many times he was still in his night clothes in bed in late morning when I came to see him. Sometimes I'd find him with his head under the pillow to snuff out the smell of Pinesol. They were able to clean his floor but not get him up for the day. Alison and I became a one-two punch: I came in the morning, she came in the afternoon after work.

Bathing became a big issue. Tracy didn't complain, but when it came time for him to take a shower, he'd go to all sorts of trouble to avoid it -- unless one specific nurse's aide was there to help. I finally got to the bottom of it. I'm sure this is common in many care facilities – some staffers are more caring than others. Some like their job better than others. Some work hard. Some avoid work. Some flat out don't like the patients. In addition to his other super sensitive reactions to light, noise, smell and taste, he developed one more: aversion to cold and inability to cope with heat. Since it was summer, the air conditioner was on. The room was cold. That bathroom was freezing. Bathrooms in care facilities are a little different than those at home: it really is a bath ROOM, not a bathtub or shower. There was no way for the room to stay warm, so someone would park him in the bathroom, turn on the shower and leave. He was so cold that he shook uncontrollably. The one aide who understood this problem made sure she had lots of towels ready for him and wrapped him up immediately after his shower. Some of the staff responsible for showering patients said he was being a baby. (In fairness to the facility, the worst staff didn't stick around long.) I've known my brother all his life. He's no baby. I made sure I was there for his showers.

We also discovered the importance of labeling all his clothes with his name. The rehabilitation center washed his clothes, but he got others' back, not his own clothes. I went through the rehabilitation center's laundry to find his belongings. I never found all of them, but we were reimbursed for the ones missing. After that, I sewed in labels with his name. It was sort of like going to summer camp.

Tracy wasn't getting time with all three therapists every day. There was always some problem: they weren't there or they couldn't stick to the schedule, or they figured Tracy should come to them and when he didn't, they went on without him. When he did go, especially for physical therapy, dizziness often got the best of him, so he was unable complete the time allotted for him. He couldn't walk a straight line or climb a set of practice stairs. He had no leg strength, no stamina, and even worse, no balance. It was big change for someone who routinely walked miles every day. The occupational therapist turned out to be a gem. Kathe had worked at the Rehabilitation Institute of Oregon and understood what they were looking for when they interviewed prospective patients. Part of her job at the rehabilitation center was to ascertain whether Tracy could re-integrate himself into the everyday world, take care of his own personal needs, cook, wash clothes, use money, and to identify whether he would need physical assistance for safety and getting around. She also was willing to conduct a home evaluation later in the summer, so we could get things taken care of before he arrived in Beaverton. We learned about front-porch ramps, grab bars and special toilet seats, and the importance of the turning radius for wheel chairs in hallways and bathrooms.

Tracy went through a series of roommates. It was a dismal failure. The facility needed to fill the other bed in his room. The other people had their own issues, but everyone in the facility was much older than Tracy. Most of his roommates, for example, were hard of hearing. One man turned the volume way up on FOX News and when he couldn't sleep in the wee hours of the night, he turned up the TV to full volume. Tracy has acute hearing ability, and he was having trouble with noise generally, so this drove him nuts. Another man wanted his wife to spend the night, and sometimes she did. That wasn't great, either.

As time went on, the routine became more predictable, and life at the Center got better. Staff and the therapists came to like Tracy. They watched him struggle with getting a handle on his balance, going from help getting into a wheelchair to wheeling the chair around the outside parking lot by himself. He graduated to using a walker inside, but he couldn't stand for long because of fatigue. He could also tip over the walker at the drop of a hat when he lost his balance.

They knew first-hand his problems with vomiting most days and nights. Early in his stay, he preferred to eat at a little table in his room. He liked having his visitors there when he ate, but his food left something to be desired. We marveled at the pureed sandwiches and a corn-like product that passed for a vegetable. However, until he could swallow food without choking, mashed-up food was the best for him.

Up to this point, it wasn't as if he had decided to be selfish, but he had no current capability to think of others. In retrospect, I marveled at his brain's ability to limit what he took in so he wasn't overwhelmed. At first he did not want to go the dining room and eat and talk with the other people in the facility. We kept trying. One day, he said he would eat lunch in the dining room. And he did, pretty much from then on. It was interesting to see the mental changes that were occurring. When he first arrived at the rehabilitation center, he had absolutely no interest in any other patients. It was almost as if it was his way of separating himself from the world in which he now found himself. He didn't consider himself like those "other" people and if he made no contact with them, they weren't "real." One jovial big guy took a liking to Tracy. Tracy finally started to warm up. When his new friend was returned to the Vet's Hospital because he'd taken a turn for the worse, Tracy was very concerned.

Tracy began to use a wheel chair to get down the hall to the therapy rooms. He worked hard to get in-and-out of it without help. He had designed an intricate overhand grappling motion that kept him steady as he got out of bed and turned to get into the chair. As long as he wasn't interrupted in the process, he did well. One day they had some kittens in the therapy room. The kittens crawled all over Tracy and he beamed. One morning, his physical therapist asked Tracy to do five leg lifts. He did six, looked at her, grinned, and said, "I gave you a bonus one!" He began to take side steps on the parallel bars and to go farther using the walker. The speech therapist really thought she could help Tracy with his swallowing and speech limitations. She and Tracy talked and agreed to try putting electrodes on his throat to zap him if his tongue got "lazy." More than once, that happened. One day, I heard a lot of laughing behind the therapy-room door. It was Tracy and the speech therapist. She had encouraged him to say the word "Fuck" because he was having real trouble using both "F's" and "K's." After looking appropriately startled, he did. Poorly at first, but louder and better with practice until they were hooting with laughter.

The high points of Tracy's days were visits from his friends. Some came and curled on the bed with him; some brought their laptops and read Facebook updates to him from other friends; one brought a Magic Bullet (a small but powerful blender) and made delicious and nutritious shakes for him. Friends brought fresh fruit and plants and a big stuffed bear. Apparently, everyone knew his love of ripe mangoes because his room overflowed with them. Others brought blankets that smelled of the ocean. Some days were pinnacles: the day Bear, Faith's eight-week old French bulldog came to give kisses and all the staff in the building came to get their share; the day Elizabeth and David, harpist and harp-builder from Lincoln City, visited and Elizabeth played her harp; and the day Chef Sharon brought and shared the gorgeous berry galette dessert she had made on a local TV show that morning – everyone knew ahead of time that a local celebrity was coming since they had tuned into the show that morning. The big deal about all that was, this was the first television Tracy had watched since his stroke. Joel, a college roommate, and his wife, Liz, brought bright new orange construction cones to serve as reminders of the cones of gelato Tracy so loved when he traveled to Italy. We still have those cones. Some made sure to ask if he'd brushed his teeth. Some took him outside to walk barefoot in the grass. Others used lotion to massage his very dry feet. Jim, a musician friend of Tracy's, and his wife, Lyn, returning from an overseas trip, came for lunch with Tracy before they even returned home. Tracy was happy his lunch stayed down, as often it didn't, but this day it behaved. Jim played his guitar and left his well-traveled hat on Tracy's head.

His friends continued to write messages to him on his Facebook page. They were his cheerleaders; caught him up on the latest gossip, and some were hilarious. After a wedding at their organic farm in August, Heidi wrote:

"...We survived another wedding yesterday/last night. Highlites (sic) from a dog's perspective include: Angel trying to get the potlatch salmon off of the barbeque...Ollie dancing to the BG's on the dance floor with all the wedding party...and...oh yes...a Piglet's perspective: lots and lots of dares to feed 'the pig' a strawberry... sort of became a rite of passage for wedding attendees!!"

Staff and the therapists got used to the large contingent of friends and family that were around Tracy all day every day. Staff at all levels commented how lucky Tracy was to have such a large and loyal following. They said it made such a difference in a patient's willingness to recover. So many of the patients had no visitors. I can't imagine spending my days alone in a place not my home with no loved ones ever coming around. Those who did get visitors often got them at mealtimes. So, mealtimes became social events. Everyone liked to hear what was going on "outside." Weather was a great topic of discussion.

Always trying to find something that Tracy liked to eat, I stopped by one of his "pre-incident" favorite restaurants, Pastini's, and picked up a Caprese salad "to go" on my way to the rehabilitation center. I had called the day before and they said they'd have it ready early the next morning. They weren't even open, but they made the salad for him. He loved it; didn't eat much of it, but he loved it.

The therapists began to involve us in Tracy's rehabilitation. Tracy was not enamored with the exercises required for speech therapy and so, the speech therapist asked for help. Tracy needed to exercise his tongue and mouth and do some speaking exercises at least twice a day. All this was extremely fatiguing. Alison helped when she visited, but for his friends, exercising his mouth and tongue must have been a whole new experience!

I kept asking Bill to come with me to the rehabilitation center to learn what was involved with physical therapy, particularly balance therapy. I asked him because if/when Tracy fell, he was the only one big enough to pick him up. Bill said he didn't understand why I wanted him to do this and he also couldn't see how he could do anything that would be of benefit. He went twice, but just stood on the sidelines. We were frustrated with each other. He has never responded well to what he perceived as being told what to do; I couldn't entice him to engage and help. I thought he just didn't want the whole thing: he didn't want to contemplate what would follow rehab. He began to say things like: "If he can't take care of himself, I'm bringing him right back here," or "I'm not going to be his nurse," or "If we weren't here, where do you think he'd end up?" After awhile, I ignored what he said. I didn't respond. I assumed part of what he was doing was just venting. I thought Alison and I could handle the physical/balance therapy when the time came. We'd have to.

Tracy had a wide variety of visitors. One day, Robin and my son, Mitch, were visiting at the same time. Robin is a very nice third-grade teacher. She made Tracy a delicious (that was Tracy's assessment) raspberry and banana smoothie. Robin called him "such a gentleman." Mitch, on the other hand, offered to bring in strippers to relieve the tedium. Another time, Sharon brought from Lincoln City two old "friends" of Tracy's to visit: her cats, Earl Grey and Crumpet. He sat in the front seat of Sharon's car and the cats crawled all over him. When she left, Sharon said he had plenty of cat hair everywhere.

Later in July, we had another meeting with staff, therapists and the social worker to discuss Tracy's condition and how we thought he was doing. The facility staff and therapists said they were "blown away" with Tracy's progress in the previous two weeks. They made a real commitment to work with him as much as he could stand to assist him regain strength, stamina and weight. They also worked on mitigating sensory overload problems, and that was helping. I asked Bill to come to this session, and he did.

Because the brain is so amazingly complex, the infinite number of possible results when blood vessels blow apart or tissue dies – as in a stroke – is a most frustrating challenge of stroke recovery. A stroke doesn't always result in sensory overload. But it did in Tracy's case. All his senses seemed to have gone crazy. Whether it was the brain, the senses or the connection between them wasn't clear. However, the result was that he smelled and tasted things he thought were awful but really weren't. It took very little light, sound, and external motion to make him curl up into a ball with his eyes shut and his hands over his ears. He suffered from cold and heat when the temperature actually was mild. He no longer knew how his body "fit" into the world around him. When asked to touch the wall while standing near it with his eyes closed, he had no idea where the wall was. His reaction when dizziness overcame him and balance eluded him was to vomit.

They dimmed the lights in the rehab workout room, took him into common areas at non-busy (and, thus, less noisy) times, and had decided to let him go without his glasses for awhile longer because he got less dizzy with them off. Once they got to know Tracy and saw how hard he was trying to recover, they all wanted to help him – really help him, not just go through the motions as they apparently had after our first group meeting. In fairness to the rehabilitationn center staff, they may experience many disappointments in their work lives and not much support from patients' family and friends. We were trying our darndest to make sure they understood how special we knew Tracy was to us.

Tracy still had bad days. He was vomiting at all times of day and night. His blood pressure was still bouncing too high and too low. Dizziness was ever-present. But when these maladies occurred, the staff checked up on him more often than required because they were genuinely concerned. When Tracy eventually left the facility, the staff said they would miss his big smile.

In early August, Bill visited Tracy and was impressed with his progress in the therapy room. About the same time, Tracy needed to see a neurologist at the Oregon Health Sciences University (OHSU) Stroke Clinic in the Hatfield Research Center in Portland as a neuro-surgery follow-up to evaluate his progress. Bill and I had done a dry-run the previous day. The occupational therapist asked if I'd drive Tracy in to the clinic because the van transports they usually used rocked wheelchair patients too much and she knew it would make Tracy very sick. We practiced getting Tracy into/out of my car and my getting the wheelchair in-and-out of the hatchback. It was heavy and awkward and I wondered if having to do this a lot was in my future. She said we passed with flying colors, so I took off with Tracy riding "shotgun" in the passenger seat for the first time in almost two months. He carried his pink pig in his lap. That's what we named the pink plastic basin that he carried with him to use in case he tossed his cookies. He'd vomited several times the previous day, but this day he was fine. The whole day was pretty overwhelming for Tracy. He liked the wind for a little while, and then asked to shut the windows. He got hot very fast, so I was glad my little car had air-conditioning. We drove the thirty-plus miles to the Portland waterfront area with his eyes mostly closed.

The Stroke Clinic medical team was efficient and appeared pleased with Tracy's progress. At my request for further clarification, the doctor said Tracy had suffered a stroke that straddled both the brain stem and cerebellum, further exacerbated by blood flooding the remainder of his brain, causing the brain to swell. Unexpected symptoms in Tracy's case included, speech problems, which normally don't occur with a brain stem/cerebellum hemorrhage, but do occur if blood causes damage in the brain's left hemisphere. We discussed continuing concerns: fluctuating blood pressure, nausea, dizziness and impaired balance aka vertigo, lack of muscle coordination, plus swallowing and speech issues. The doctor was very concerned about pinpointing the cause of Tracy's blood-presssure fluctuations. He said blood pressure is controlled by the heart and the kidneys, and if it wasn't controlled, Tracy could suffer a repeat "incident." We talked about changing medication, hopefully lessening the dosage and fewer medications, to discover whether that might help quell the substantial side effects Tracy was suffering. Side effects included dizziness and nausea. I asked how we could tell what was stroke-related and what was a side effect of medication. The doctor wrote notes to the rehabilitation facility physician recommending that he review all blood-pressure medications and call in a specialist to help determine the cause and location of the fluctuation. Finally, I asked about a referral to the Rehabilitation Institute of Oregon (RIO) and whether the neurologist would make the referral, which he did.

After this visit, Tracy was exhausted and so appreciated this message from his sweet friend, Robin:

"King Arthur – Tracy

Dear Tracy,

I am sitting here this morning, reading Wendy's update on your appointment at OHSU. And I can't help thinking of you now, with your dragons to slay – the blood pressure dragon and the vertigo dragon especially. And I can't help thinking of you with your tests to pass – the tests you overcome everyday in your rehabilitation and therapy sessions, and all the tests that you overcome just navigating through your day.

"I am imagining you as King Arthur. And all the rest of us are Knights of the Round Table. You couldn't see us all at your OHSU appointment yesterday, but we were there. All circled around your spirit, waiting for news of which dragons to slay, and which victories to celebrate. I think that only King Arthur knows for sure who/where/what will be his Merlin and his

Excalibur. Maybe some magical alchemy of fruit smoothies, doctors, nurses, medicines, therapies… Maybe King Arthur's supporters and Knights. I only know that King Arthur will find Merlin to guide him and Excalibur to help him fight his battles. He already has a heart full of strength and courage enough for all of us.

"I'm not sure that I can compare Forest Grove to Camelot. But at least I can say that your Knights are spread all across the land, fighting for you with our love and our hope and any small things that we can do. You are in our hearts continually. We miss you. We love you. And any swords we can muster are at the ready. Maybe you can imagine us all out here, fighting beside you in spirit while you are slaying dragons and celebrating victories. Just look back over the incredible obstacles you have already overcome. I am so proud of you, my friend. Of everything you have already accomplished, and all that you are going to accomplish. I can't wait to see you again next week. All my love… "

The same day, Kelly wrote:

"…I look forward to the fall coming and time passing because I know it means you will be making more progress. Soon I will begin making glass again and your spirit will be in every piece and I will bring my favorite ones to share with you, like I always do. Thank you so much for so many gifts you have given us and continue to give us. You have taught us about living and what is important in this life…"

Tracy was a work in progress. The doctor changed medications again based on current results and tests taken at OHSU, trying to see what fit best for him. Staff tried to space out dosages (some before, some after breakfast, for example) but Tracy still had to take some of them four times a day. They decided to try Dramamine for the vertigo/balance/dizziness. He still had daily blood-pressure fluctuation and episodes of vomiting. They continued to try to determine the source of the blood-pressure fluctuations. They knew vomiting was a direct result of the type of stroke he had and everyone hoped that with time, healing in the part of his brain that was so damaged would eventually end the nausea. Even though not medically trained, I worked with the medical staff on adjusting medication. They appreciated my input, especially since I saw him much more than they did. Lay people can, indeed, have input for their loved ones even in the murky field of pharmaceuticals.

In mid-August, staff told me I could take Tracy on a mini-vacation to one of our favorite local restaurants, Murray Hill Cafe, so I called Bill to join us, loaded Tracy and the wheel chair in my car and off we went. After we parked at the restaurant, I unloaded the wheel chair and locked its wheels by Tracy's car door. He stood up, turned, sat down by himself, and then wheeled himself into the restaurant. The restaurant staff applauded. Tracy ordered a Greek omelette, ate a bit more than half, and drank a glass of orange juice. We enjoyed the lovely day, the view over the lake, and good conversation. Then, he wheeled himself back to the car and got in. As I started to drive away, he threw-up his breakfast. We were treating this behavior with increasing aplomb. It had become not a big thing – as long as the pink pig was handy.

A week later, we kept another appointment with another doctor in Portland, this time a physiatrist, a physician with a specialty in rehabilitation who could recommend (or not recommend) Tracy's admittance to the Rehabilitation Institute of Oregon (RIO). The doctor asked Tracy to walk down a hallway by himself. My heart was in my mouth because I just knew he'd fall into one of the cabinets along the wall. He did, but the doctor was right there and kept him from going to the floor. Tracy made it farther than I expected. The doctor was impressed with Tracy's progress, and believed there was more progress to be made, so he recommended that Tracy be accepted at RIO for inpatient rehabilitation. Bill, Tracy and I met at Pastini's, an often-frequented restaurant, to celebrate, and this time Tracy didn't toss his cookies.

About this time, Bill and I had a discussion about Bill's beloved, but aging Toyota pickup. I was willing to ride in the tiny backseat for years, whenever we traveled as a threesome, because I was the smallest. We realized that Tracy would be coming to live at our house at some point, and we would need more room for equipment, as well as a body, and they wouldn't all fit in the pickup's backseat. I asked him to try out a Toyota Prius, a gas-electric hybrid car. If it didn't suit him, I wouldn't push him to get it. He drove to the dealership "just to look," and after checking how a wheelchair/walker would fit, he came home with a red, four-door Prius hatchback he promptly named "Baby." So much for Bill not being "engaged" in what was going on in our lives. In retrospect, I think this was another example of him seeing a solution to a problem that he could do something about, so he did.

Tracy was spending early mornings wheeling himself around the parking lot in his wheelchair. He was out-and-about much more: Kelly, and her children, Dylan and Rowan, brought a Thai meal to share with Tracy.

One lovely weekend afternoon in late August, several of his friends put together a lunch out at the local McMenamin's Pub where Bill and I joined them all, bringing Tracy. Jane, photographer and former studio-mate of Tracy's and her husband, Scott, the crazy man who moved so many of Tracy's belongings, had offered to give him a ride on the back of one of their motorcycles, and he laughed.

We brought Tracy home for a weekend to watch his beloved Oregon Ducks in their first football game of the 2011 season. Tracy and I also spent part of an afternoon at near-by Jackson Bottom Wetlands, looking for eagles. We didn't stay long because the motion of trying to follow the eagles' flight triggered nausea.

I took him for his very first pedicure. He was fascinated by the art being painted onto the nails of the young lady sitting next to him – an Oregon State University (OSU) Beaver who loved their orange and black colors. Her nails were blossoming with white flowers on an orange background. He was modest in his own choice of color that day – just clear polish. In subsequent pedicure visits, he chose silver, aqua green and royal purple.

Tracy sought to keep his spirits up while he waited the interminable wait to hear if/when he was going to move on. Waiting is hard for anyone. He had worked very hard to get to the level he needed to "graduate" to the next level and in his new, more literal self, he was ready so everyone else should be, too. It would be a full month of waiting before he could go to the next level. The waiting was not for medical reasons, but rather for insurance staff to determine whether they wanted him at RIO.

Alison and I tried all sorts of cheerleading acts to help Tracy keep up his spirits. He became more depressed by the day. I was rattling every cage I could find, up-and-down the state bureaucracy to find what the holdup was. I spent much time on hold and speaking to voice mail but one "real" person I talked with suggested that we just wait to see what Medicaid/Oregon Health Plan decided and if we didn't like it, we could appeal it. I wondered if this was an indication of the slimy junction between healthcare and insurance. An appeal would probably take more than a year. I believed that we didn't have even months. Tracy responded best to daily intervention and activity, just like most stroke victims do and waiting was positively detrimental to his staying on a positive course. I called the Governor's Office. Each time his staff referred me to someone else and I was either put on hold or got a voicemail. I called the Governor's Office again... four times. Finally, I got someone willing to look into why the decision was taking so long -- and to call me back with an answer. All these days, Tracy got quieter and slower. He began shutting down. His doctor at the rehabilitation center said stroke victims often suffered from depression, and he suggested putting Tracy on anti-depressants. I resisted until all his therapists told me that he needed some help, and that his taking anti-depressants would not affect his RIO application. They also suggested we begin the process of finding a counselor to go along with the medication.

During this long wait, Tracy received his regular contingent of visitors from Lincoln City, and he received this great message from his photographer friend, Jane:

"Hi Tracy – It was wonderful to see you today. You look so good! I can see as each week goes by, how much healthier you are getting. And what blows me away is how, in spite of your anxiety and eagerness to get out of there and over to RIO, you still have a great sense of humor. You are so grounded about this. And I love your excuse for everything else: "Well, I had a stroke!" Yeah, you did, but I love how you don't let that stop you from moving ahead. Both Matt and I agree that not only are you an inspiration, but you are a comfort to those of us who love you. We are all lucky people. So, my friend, Matt and I are off to the civilized wilds of Europe. You will be with us in spirit, both metaphysically and materially speaking. If your ears are burning, know that we are sitting somewhere in Paris, Venice, Tuscany or Rome, toasting you with a glass of very good Cab, wishing you were with us. See you in a month!"

(Lest anyone be concerned, there are two "Matts" in this story. This is not Tracy's Matt, but Jane's son, Matt!)

A post on Facebook from an old friend who had just heard about Tracy's event was a reminiscence of time they had spent together that, when I read it to Tracy, made him laugh: *"...Remember our trip to the Alvord (Desert in southeastern Oregon) and the day we had to flee the water blowing across the playa in the midst of brewing that infamous "Band-Aid Beer"...Ha!"* I got a very different perspective of my little brother when his friends chimed in with "Remember the time when..." It came to me that he was wild, free, loony, fearless, a lover of life, very inventive, and he had a great love of high speed.

On Facebook another post: *"...Sounds like RIO is a great place for Tracy and I wish him all the best. I am convinced he will work hard and make wonderful progress. Keeping you in my prayers. I'm just a caring former neighbor. :-)"*

While many of Tracy's visitors came to see him, returned home and wrote of their day with him so others would catch up on the day's news, many others just visited faithfully and didn't write about it. All their visits nourished Tracy's soul.

Chapter 7:
Not Everyone Makes it at Rehab Boot Camp …

In late September, 2011, Tracy rolled into RIO, a division of the Legacy/Good Samaritan Hospital Network in Portland. He was there for twelve days.

When Tracy left the rehabilitation center, the staff gave him a going-away party complete with cake, and he received many cards from the people who had cared for him. He was deposited into my car via their wheel chair. I felt naked because we left without the wheel chair. I took him to RIO close to downtown Portland and they provided a wheel chair in the hospital lobby. We ventured to the fifth Floor and settled Tracy into his room, where he met his roommate, who was eating a pizza and told Tracy he didn't know what he was in for.

We were asked to provide comfortable clothing suitable for therapy, which started that afternoon. Staff welcomed Tracy and asked if he was ready to get very, very tired. He would work in forty-five-minute increments, not the fifteen-twenty minute increments he was used to at the rehab center. The work sessions were separated by short rests, but there were double sessions daily: a set of three in the morning and three in the afternoon. There also were extensive medical work-ups, tests and assessments of his physical and mental condition. The next day, I brought the clothing they asked for and began the laundry run. Every other day I brought clean clothes and took home dirty ones to wash.

The first session of each therapy (the now-familiar Triumverate of Therapies: physical/balance, occupational and speech) was spent in assessing where Tracy was on a continuum of totally independent to totally dependent/needing assistance. The first morning I found him lying exhausted on top of his bed, having finished two of the three sets of therapies earlier that morning. He didn't even get under the covers. I dragged the blanket over him because he was cold. Several minutes later, the next therapist came to get him. Tracy looked at me and said, "Not sure I can do this." I told him it was the hardest thing he would ever do, but that everyone thought he was capable of becoming more independent and this was the best way to do it. He sighed and then got up and left with the therapist. Tracy's roommate stayed in bed while I arranged Tracy's clothes in the closet so it would be easy for him to get them when needed. I asked his roommate how long he had been there and he said "a couple of days." I asked if he had therapy every day and he said, "I'm supposed to, but I can't handle it."

Tracy returned almost an hour later, just in time for lunch. He could barely hold his eyes open. He didn't want to eat because he was so tired. I annoyed him persistently until he picked at the food before falling asleep. The next round of therapy began in early afternoon. The therapist woke him. Shortly after that, I also left, stopping at the front desk to get their assessment of how Tracy was settling in. They said he was struggling a lot with fatigue and exhaustion but that was common for people who had strokes. Otherwise, he was behaving as they expected.

I called that evening after dinner to check on Tracy. He was sleeping. Because of his balance issues, they pulled up the rails on his bed so he wouldn't fall out. It also meant he couldn't get out of bed on his own; they were being cautious after reading the notes from the rehabilitation center.

In the days to come, I returned each day to see how things were going. He had a new roommate. I was able to observe Tracy in therapy which was an eye opener, surprising me as to the intense and extensive nature of the work. For example, the physical therapists worked with him on expanding his use of the wheelchair, walker and cane; and they introduced a gait strap wrapped around his waist, where he walked independently, but his companion was close at hand with a hand wrapped around the gait strap at Tracy's back. I learned to walk with him using the gait strap. Without a tight hold, he would fall over like a tree trunk, most often backwards, toward his left. Walking with the gait strap was very different from the other assistance tools he was using. He had nothing to hang on to, so he had no immediate reference point. At this time, the hope was to make it possible for him to navigate at our house using the wheelchair and later, hopefully, the walker. Much depended on if he learned new ways to balance.

The occupational therapist was great. He helped determine the state of Tracy's mental judgment. The degree to which Tracy could become independent rested in large part on how well he could make appropriate, safe decisions and it got to be a standing joke between them: he was not to leave any burners lit on the stove when he left a room, and no firearms were to be used in carrying out any decisions. Tracy, the ultimate peacemaker, thought this was very funny. Not so funny; it seems that many people who suffer strokes lose their ability to act safely. Determining how they can live their lives safely and appropriately is a big clue as to the kind of post-stroke life they can lead. The occupational therapist also was instrumental in helping us obtain a handicap-parking sticker from the Oregon Department of Motor Vehicles and complete an application to get bus transport after Tracy moved to our house.

A word about occupational therapy and occupational therapists. I pretty well understood the role of physical therapists and speech therapists. I could see how important their work was in getting individuals back on their feet and communicating. When I first heard about occupational therapists, I had no idea of their value. I mistakenly thought they helped people pick out a new occupation, and then I thought they helped with basic stuff like how to cook and clean and go shopping – basic necessities but not requiring the training that a physical or speech therapist needed. I was very wrong. All three disciplines are incredibly necessary in knitting together a new life for a person forever changed by some massive head trauma. The judgment of an occupational therapist as to the mental and emotional stability of a patient is critical as to whether they achieve an independent life style.

Five days after Tracy arrived at RIO, a team meeting was called with the lead doctor, the three therapists, the social worker, Tracy, and me. They complimented Tracy on being one of their "star" patients, saying he would get the Smiles Award when he graduated, which they expected to be eight days later on his birthday, October 6. Their assessment concluded that in addition to the first (hemorrhagic) stroke he had in the cerebellar region of his brain and the damage that it had caused, a brain scan showed damaging evidence of three additional clotting strokes: one in the right frontal lobe, which affects short and mid-term memory, and two in the left parietal (side) lobe, affecting language. (That cleared up a major question in my mind. Immediately after his first stroke, he was still able to speak and string words together. It was after the subsequent strokes that his real difficulties began with language.) He was still struggling with vision/balance and vertigo. When he used his right hand to draw (which they had asked him to do on a big board while standing because it simulated the way he had painted in his studio) straight away he became dizzy and nauseated. He fell sideways or into the board. When they asked him to read or write, the same phenomenon occurred. They determined that eye movement triggered vertigo and nausea. He was making great strides learning to independently care for himself, but he needed someone close at hand because of his continuing balance problems. The suggestion was made that although he always had used a hand razor for shaving, for the foreseeable future it would be best for him to use an electric razor. I bought an electric razor and brought it to RIO the next day.

The speech therapist played a big role in the assessment. She said Tracy was struggling with a number of intertwined issues like dysphagia, a condition where throat and mouth muscles are weakened by a stroke. The connection is damaged between the brain and these muscles. In Tracy's case, he struggled not to choke on food, but choking on water was his real issue. She worked to teach Tracy various "tricks" to help him swallow water without choking. As with many other activities, as long as he was not distracted and could retain focus, he did better. He had difficulty remembering linear instructions, but they were trying ways to assist him with his short-term memory. As for speech, he struggled with speaking, reading, writing, and word comprehension and retrieval. These functions originate in different parts of the brain, and, therefore, having multiple difficulties is more challenging to address. Specifically, he suffered from expressive and retrieval aphasia and ataxic dysarthria.

I was ignorant of the amazing complexity of speech. I heard more words that I took home to study: Dysphagia, expressive aphasia, retrieval aphasia, ataxic dysarthria, articulation, phonation, and prosody. Aphasia is a disorder that results from damage to sections of the brain controlling language. Expressive aphasia involves conveying thoughts through speech or writing. A person knows what he wants to say, but cannot find the words needed. Retrieval aphasia involves difficulty finding a name of something and not being able to put words to an idea. Often a person tends to recover skills in language comprehension more completely than those skills involving expression. All types of dysarthria affect the articulation of consonants, causing the slurring of speech, and in very severe cases, vowels also may be distorted.

Tracy slurred his words and sometimes spoke with what therapists call a "wet voice," almost gargling as if his mouth was full of water while he attempted to speak. Ataxic dysarthria is a disorder due to damage to the cerebellar control circuit. Tracy's particular challenges involved articulation, prosody: placing equal and excessive stress on all syllables spoken, and phonation. Sometimes his speech was explosive with excessive loudness. It's important to know how this difficulty manifests itself because, in the outside world, if someone came upon Tracy who didn't recognize that he'd had a stroke, that person might well conclude that Tracy was drunk and take actions accordingly. That would be unhelpful.

Finally, the team talked about blood pressure. The medical team modified his medications and was using his time at RIO to assess his reaction. It was aggressive therapy in a closely watched environment. They wanted to solve the persistent instability and spikes of his blood pressure. The range it traveled was far too great and they wanted better control, specifically since his next step was living outside a medical or care facility. They had tentatively settled on four blood-pressure medications, three at full strength, and one slightly less, that they believed might be the best "cocktail" for the time being. The doctor emphasized her concern, going forward, for Tracy. She said that one side effect of chronically elevated blood pressure, which Tracy had, was hardening of the arteries and that condition statistically increased the potential of another stroke. The team emphasized a lifestyle that included as little stress as possible, a healthy diet, finding and keeping an appropriate weight and regular exercise. They felt his chosen profession as an artist was a great one for the life ahead of him: it was something he loved, something he had done well, and something that allowed unlimited creativity. He would have challenges controlling his fine motor skills, fatigue from standing, nausea from eye movement – especially up-and-down across a large canvas -- but it was a purpose for life.

All along, the Lincoln City Contingent kept in touch. Tracy was so exhausted during his days at RIO, that although he appreciated their thinking of him, he asked that they not travel the more than one-hundred miles just to watch him sleep – if they caught him in his room at all. The first Sunday in October, RIO gave us a "day pass" and I brought Tracy home on a glorious but cold afternoon to watch his grand-nephew, Trenton, play "Fall Ball" (baseball) in Hillsboro. Being outside exhausted him, but I noted he really tried to focus on Trenton when he was either up to bat or playing the field. When I took him back to RIO, he leaned back in the seat with his eyes closed, but smiled when I asked him if he'd had a good time. I was getting more used to the routine of transporting Tracy. Each time he rode in the car, we took blankets, a jacket, scarf and hat (even though he hated hats because they hurt his head. Later, Sharon, a chef of many talents, knitted him a soft purple hat he loved); dark glasses, a box of tissues, a clean rag and towel and the handicap-parking sticker for the car. At first, we took the pink pig but one of my bridge-playing "sisters," a regular hospital volunteer at eighty-eight years old who had suffered her own traumatic brain injury years before, brought me a small, rolled up and much less obvious "throw-up bag." I bought a supply, and Bill and I learned to carry several in both our cars, and when Tracy traveled with someone else. Soon we also learned the value of a handicap-parking sticker: it went with Tracy in whatever vehicle he traveled.

Near the end of Tracy's stay at RIO, another far-away college friend, Bruce, sent a great email asking how Tracy was doing with his drawing. That was a question on everyone's mind, even those of us who saw him regularly. Bruce wrote that he did a little woodworking, and that he had made Tracy a sketching pencil "... BUT I do not want to send it at an inappropriate time... I want to encourage him to pick up his tools again but I don't want it to be a frustration for him. I don't want good intentions to come off as inconsiderate, ill informed, or unsympathetic. Being a couple of thousand miles away has its drawbacks..."

What a sensitive and astute observation! Bruce reminded me that Tracy was best man at his wedding and that they, Tracy and Bruce, had danced together at the reception for no other reason than to "have a good time and to celebrate. When we finished, my mom asked if we had done that before! Well, we hadn't but her question made me laugh ... we were just having a good time." It would be a long time before that pencil came to Tracy and even longer before he tried sketching again.

The last few days at RIO were a whirlwind. I made sure our house was ready for Tracy and received final instructions from the medical staff and the therapists. I began looking for therapists convenient to our home so he could continue to make progress on all fronts. I didn't want any regression. On the morning Tracy was discharged, we almost had a hiccup. RIO rules would not allow him to be discharged if he didn't have a wheel chair. The Oregon Health Plan would not pay the wheel chair provider for a wheel chair used at RIO. I couldn't take home a wheel chair from RIO. I also couldn't take the wheel chair provided for Tracy to go home until someone agreed to pay for it. It was a stand-off and neither side would budge. In frustration, I wrote a check to the wheel chair provider for the first month's rent for the chair so I could get Tracy out of RIO and home. The whole medical-equipment issue and payment for same would return to cause trouble in the future.

As before when Tracy left OHSU for the rehabilitation center, I thought the time he had with them wasn't nearly enough to help with everything he needed. But again, look what was accomplished: RIO had done wonders and the most important part was they opened our eyes to the real possibilities of what Tracy could achieve. They also were very realistic in what it would take to get him there. Most notably, Alison and I came away absolutely sure we could make "this" work for Tracy.

Although woven together into our family's fabric, everyone within the family reacted differently to Tracy's stroke. Right after the first paroxysm of shock, we clung together. We reached out to far-flung family members with whom we were not in regular contact.

Early on, although I couldn't actually see it, I just knew a long road lay ahead filled with curves and hills. What I didn't know was what was at roads-end, how long it would take to get there, and whether I could survive an ending I feared.

My family propped me up. When I needed unconditional support, my daughter was right there. She had her own life, her own demons, and her own problems. She was at my side during the terrifying first days and for many months afterward. I asked my son to take charge of Tracy's beloved 4-Runner, Luna. To this day, Luna stays at his house waiting for Tracy. Two of my three grandchildren visited Tracy as often as their schedules allowed. Other family from across the country checked in, sent best wishes, visited, and when the time was right, Tracy would visit them.

I save a special place in my heart for Bill, my husband, because our life during this time became complicated. I know he loves me very deeply. Otherwise, he'd have been gone. I think that when some people accomplish getting their lives arranged just the way they like, they resist change – particularly change they don't like. Bill would say, I believe, that he very much tried to help, but I also believe that he worked hard to hang on to his old life. More than once since Tracy's incident, Bill had said he might just leave. I told him he had to do what he had to do, but I hoped he'd come back. The week before Tracy came "home," Bill flew to the Chicago area for a week to see his daughter, her family, and a longtime friend. He got home the night before Tracy came "home." A week after that, Bill left again, this time for California for another week to see friends and family. I was happy he was taking these trips because I thought he needed to refresh his perspective. I hoped he'd come back. He did. He said he thought of staying away, but he couldn't. He loved me too much.

Tracy "graduated" from RIO and came "home" on his birthday, October 6: three months and 16 days after his "event" at the gym in Lincoln City. It was a full day getting him settled in, celebrating his birthday, filling several prescriptions – and finding a big pill box to hold them all -- plus watching the Oregon Ducks on TV. We watched football, but I kept the TV sound low because unexpected noise, such as crowds erupting into cheers at some spectacular play, still made Tracy jump. Actually, Bill and I watched football and Tracy slept in his favorite easy chair. Watching TV or anything that moved nauseated him. He did O.K. getting up-and-down the hall in his wheelchair to the bathroom. Earlier in the summer, based on the input from the rehabilitation center's occupational therapist who had conducted a "home visit" at my request, and with top-notch help from our friend, Paul, the contractor, we had "Tracy-proofed" the house. In the bathroom, we took up all the rugs, installed a special toilet seat with sides and added a shower bench. We streamlined his bedroom (located next to the room where I slept), adding open closet shelves and shelves on the wall over a desk that accommodated his wheel chair and that had a few of his books, pictures, computer, and art work on it to remind him of his previous life. We had to be sure there was room for his wheel chair to move around including getting him to his bed. And, Paul built an appropriately angled ramp to the front door so we could get the wheel chair into the house.

Tracy would live with us for the next twenty-three months.

Chapter 8:
A Whole New World:
The Care Track and the Official Track...
and the Paperwork that Keeps Everything Afloat

If someone were to ask me now what I thought was the most heroic job in today's world, my answer, hands down, would be caregiver. I've backed into this conclusion, having no idea what I was getting into, and I base it on the many examples I saw during this time with Tracy. I had no real idea what a caregiver did. As an old joke says, "And now I are one."

There are the obvious duties of physical care. The less tangible but maybe greater burdens are mysterious, frustrating and overwhelming. The role of advocate is major because if a caregiver is unable to put on and wear the cloak of advocacy, the likelihood of success at the end of the day for either them or their loved one is very poor. Advocacy requires total and fearless commitment. The role changes based on the situation. Caregivers have to be able to do just about anything, with few tools, less knowledge, and often in very little time. With stellar exceptions, I saw that most caregivers are women and most of the women are of a "certain age" who are inexperienced with hoisting heavy equipment (e.g., a wheelchair into the trunk of a car). Most have raised their families and are in the time of their lives when they think they can slow down, take a breath, look around, and see what they'd like to do for pleasure. All caregivers have a "day when everything changed."

As Bill and I were sitting in the waiting room at the Oregon Health Sciences University Hospital (OHSU) and my brother, Tracy, was in recovery from surgery the morning after he was Life Flighted in from Lincoln City, we were visited by a very nice lady representing the business arm of OHSU. She introduced herself as Jackie, a Medicaid Specialist from Financial and Medicaid Services. She had some papers in her hand. She asked us some questions, determined that I was the relative of the person involved, and so she directed more questions to me: did Tracy have a wife? Children? A POLST (Physician Orders for Life-Sustaining Treatment)? An advance directive? Medical insurance? Was there a Power of Attorney? A Health Care Representative? The answer to all her questions (after determining what some of them meant) was, "no." I told her I was his closest living relative.

She said that since Tracy was unable to fill out the necessary forms, I needed to complete them so they could be submitted to the State of Oregon as well as to OHSU's business/credit office. There was one form for OHSU. It was six pages. There was an application for Medicaid benefits from the Oregon Department of Human Services Seniors and People with Disabilities. It was 12 pages. There was another four-page form from the same folks called "Authorization for Use and Disclosure of Information," that needed filling out.

Jackie said it was very important for us to figure a way to obtain a Health Care Power of Attorney and a Durable Unlimited Power of Attorney that would cover the financial arena. Without the Health Care Power of Attorney, the medical establishment could not give me any information about Tracy's status, treatment, or prognosis, and I would have no control over what happened to him. Without a Financial Power of Attorney, I would be unable to get any financial information from banks, credit-card companies, even utility and cable-TV companies so there would be no way to understand or control his financial situation. The State wanted me to give them information about Tracy, but they could not give me any information about what they did with that information if I didn't sign their "Authorization Form."

I looked at the list of items needed for the forms: family information, proof of residence, proof of identification, proof of citizenship, health-insurance cards, a copy of his Social Security card, policies and premium statements, Power of Attorney papers, employment and all other income information, itemization of Tracy's total assets including current checking/savings account statements, life and burial-insurance policies, real-estate documents including any transactions in the last sixty months, retirement funds including Individual Retirement Accounts (IRAs), and vehicle(s). They also wanted all current shelter and medical costs. My eyes glazed over long before I finished reading the list.

I had no idea what the answers were to most of these questions. Worse, the answers were more than hundred miles away somewhere in Tracy's house. I couldn't go to Lincoln City while he was in such a precarious medical condition, but how else could I get the information they needed? Ten days later, I was in Lincoln City trying to find some answers to their questions. While I was back in Beaverton, his friends had driven his car home and put it into the garage; emptied his mailbox and brought everything into the house; turned off a light; and watered his plants. He had, after all, left his house one afternoon just to exercise at the gym. He expected to be back in a couple of hours.

Tracy worked part-time at Volta Glass Gallery in Lincoln City. Kelly made sure his paycheck was deposited into his Credit Union checking account. Lincoln City is a small town. Word of Tracy's "event" traveled like wildfire. Everyone knew something awful had happened. I stopped at the credit union on my way into town and asked the question that I would be asking a lot: "What do you need from me so I can get access to his account?" The answer was uniform: Power of Attorney. Or, we could wait for the State to handle everything (a few years at least down the road). The costs would be unbelievable and Tracy would never recover financially. Once I got to his house, I went to his office and went through what I could find of his personal papers and financial records. Tracy always was well organized, but I found very little paperwork. Apparently, he did almost everything online. I was stumped. That's when I contacted Harry. Harry had just graduated from high school. He had immersed himself into all things computer/internet since he was age 12 and Tracy had helped him build his first website.

On that first visit to Lincoln City, I gathered what information I could find that helped answer the questions on the forms from OHSU and the State Department of Human Services and Oregon Health Plan. I knew I could piece together his income/expenses information, but I needed time with his computer to determine how he did his books. While in Lincoln City, Harry helped me get it.

Before I could complete the Power of Attorney, I didn't know how many bills of Tracy's needed payment. I didn't know who his creditors were. I just knew that as each day passed, bills kept accruing and payments were being made on autopilot. I had to get into the driver's seat of this moving train before it crashed and burned.

In addition to a small studio at his house, Tracy painted in a studio in town. As noted before, I talked with his landlord and worked out an arrangement whereby some of Tracy's exceptional friends would take down the studio, bring everything to Tracy's garage, and thus end the rental arrangement.

I visited all the creditors I could identify, told them what I hoped to do, and came back home two days later. I went right on to the hospital to see Tracy.

In the meantime, I asked Jackie from OHSU's Financial and Medicaid Department to describe the exact forms needed for the Power of Attorney. She gave us that information and when I was in Lincoln City, Bill found blank forms at Office Depot. We still had a problem: Tracy had to be awake enough to sign the forms – and to know what he was signing. And, two witnesses were required when Tracy was awake and able to sign.

Help arrived at just the right time in the form of another set of marvelous friends: Long-time friends Allan and Carol who came from Reno to see Tracy. The day after Tracy moved from the Neurosciences ICU to the Kohler Acute Care Unit, we had the forms completed except for signatures. I asked Tracy if he was O.K. with me representing him, and said we needed the forms signed so I could act on his behalf for medical and financial reasons. He understood and nodded "yes." The Notary Public at OHSU was put on notice that we would need her, and Tracy's friends were in the room visiting. We called the Notary but we weren't sure how long Tracy would be awake. She was delayed. We all left Tracy's room to let him rest. She went to the room, saw him sleeping and started to leave. We caught up with her, explained what was happening, and she was very concerned that Tracy understand what was being asked of him. I asked her to come back into the room and be the judge. I woke Tracy. He wasn't very chipper, but I asked him to sit up because we needed him to sign the papers we had talked about. He said "O.K." I introduced him to the Notary and said she wanted to ask him a few questions. He nodded. She was satisfied that he knew what he was signing. I showed her his driver's license. His friends attested that they knew it was Tracy and that he was the person signing the form. I appreciated that the Notary was being careful. But I was glad when the forms were all complete.

Even before obtaining the Power of Attorney, I called the local office of Social Security. My new mentor, Jackie, suggested we apply immediately for Social Security Disability for Tracy since the medical reports regarding his situation indicated that, from today's perspective, it was unlikely he would recover sufficiently to earn an independent living. I understood the reason for the suggestion and she made it in a soothing, calm way. But the enormity of what was happening – that Tracy might never again create art or live independently – made me just sob. Then I quit blubbering and made the earliest appointment possible with Social Security: two weeks away. That appointment created a cascade of forms and lists of required information: proof of income for the past two years, proof of medical disability, his birth certificate, his witnessed signature on a document called "Authorization to Disclose Information to the Social Security Administration (SSA)" – his signature. Right. It wouldn't look anything like his previous signature. Was that O.K.? I began gathering the documentation I needed for the appointment.

The next project was to complete the two sets of forms for the OHSU Financial and Medicaid Services Office, the State Department of Human Services and the Oregon Health Plan. By faxing copies of the Power of Attorney forms, I was able to get Tracy's current financial information and, thus, complete the required paperwork. I had another challenge: income verification and business expenses. Tracy was employed part-time at the Glass Gallery. I got copies of check stubs from his employer, no problem. The challenge was, he was also a self-employed artist who was represented by four galleries. Additionally, he painted commissions (art installations for people who contracted with him directly). His "event" occurred just prior to the end of the second quarter. He had completed neither an Income Statement nor a Profit and Loss Statement for the first half of the year. I found the contact information for the four art galleries who represented him, called them and asked that they send me amounts paid to Tracy for specific pieces sold in 2011 and the dates they paid him for the sales. The galleries responded quickly.

Lest anyone mistakenly think Tracy was a high-flying artist with lots of money, please remember there had been a lengthy economic downturn for the past several years prior to his "event." When people don't have jobs or when "things are tight," they don't purchase much in the way of art. He was hanging on financially by the skin of his teeth. I went through as much paperwork as I could find to make sure I hadn't missed anything.

I turned in the forms to OHSU and the State of Oregon twenty-two days after Tracy had his stroke. By that time, bills had arrived from Lincoln City Hospital, Lincoln City Ambulance and Life Flight. Considering that Tracy had no health insurance, those bills were astronomical. They would be enough to choke someone who had health insurance. I felt badly about

Tracy's lack of health insurance, but as a "starving artist," I'm guessing he determined that he could not afford the monthly premiums. I also would guess that if he had found something wrong, he would not have been able to afford treatment costs. Should he have had health insurance? Obviously, as it turned out. He's not the only American who has chosen to pay some other bill or buy food instead of health insurance. I remember a woman I knew who worked at the U.S. Department of Labor in Washington, D.C., who held a very popular lottery every other Friday. It was payday and people bet substantial sums of money on which bills she would pay with her current paycheck. Tracy didn't reckon with genetics: our mom suffered from high-blood pressure for years. I knew that, but I'm not sure he did. His solution to having too little to purchase health insurance and medications was to try to live a healthy life, eat well and exercise. If he had not, I doubt he would have survived his "event." From all appearances, he was very healthy and a great example of why high blood pressure is called the silent killer.

Jackie, now my mentor-guru at OHSU, had looked over the forms and the information I gathered thus far and pinpointed one problem: his Individual Retirement Account (IRA). It would be cashed out and applied toward his mounting medical bills. I remembered how hard he worked to save the $2,000 placed into that account. And it was disappearing in a poof just like that, leaving him with just Social Security when he retired. But I could see no alternative. I contacted TRowePrice, explained the situation, and they took care of everything.

Next I went to the Social Security office, documents in hand, less than one month after Tracy's "event." I met with a very no-nonsense lady speaking clearly but with a Russian accent. She never smiled. She was as close to a drill sergeant as I've ever met. As she moved through the appointment, and in subsequent dealings I had with her, she remained very no-nonsense, but also so very helpful. She was unfazed about someone applying for someone else's disability, and explained plainly that once I had given her all the documentation and information requested, Tracy seemed likely to receive Social Security Disability. She said if he were medically approved, he would be eligible six months from the date of his "event," with his first check arriving a month later. The amount was small, but appreciated. However, I didn't see how anyone could live on it. That was a problem for another day. She also suggested that I do two more things -- complete a form called "Appointment of Representative" signed by Tracy and me so I could provide information to, and receive information from, Social Security on his behalf – and I should apply right away for Supplemental Security Income (SSI) which, if he were eligible, would kick in after a one-month waiting period and fill-in until he could collect disability payments. Of course, the documentation was a little different along with another set of forms, and income-eligibility requirements were more restrictive. So I left that meeting with more tasks to complete. I filled out the Social Security forms that night, had Tracy sign them the next day (one month precisely from his "event") and I returned them to the local Social Security office.

Over the next several months I received many more sets of forms and requests for additional information. Social Security doesn't recognize a Power of Attorney. Instead, they wanted different forms: one for me to give on, one for me to receive information from them. They dated regarding income during the time the application was More than once I received a cover letter saying if I didn't his application would be ruled on immediately and that e averse to Tracy's cause. I kept sending completed forms "live" officials. Finally, I reached a nice lady who knew what e said not to worry about the form letters I received. She it until September when she would send me what was needed. She also said she was the one who would make the preliminary ruling on Tracy's application and nothing would be done for three months. She was waiting on medical reports indicating his condition since his condition hadn't yet stabilized sufficiently to make any long-term medical predictions.

Tracy was approved for Medicaid/Oregon Health Plan one week later, which, I was told, was pretty quick. I had called a few times to see if they needed any additional information. That was my way of "checking" to assure myself that things were moving along. There were some questions about his income. It's hard for salaried people to understand the finances of a self-employed artist who doesn't receive a regular paycheck. They were non-plussed that he didn't earn a regular amount each month. I explained how it worked and then the person I was talking with understood. Later, I got used to re-explaining everything to new people who called. I rarely got calls from the same person; it was always someone else and that meant we had to once again start from the beginning.

Tracy was transferred to the rehabilitation center a week prior to the State's approval of his application. But when we visited the Center, we told them we had applied for aid and they seemed confident there would not be a problem. OHSU also did not seem concerned. We were never pressured by either facility for payment. On the other hand, the bills from Lincoln City Hospital, their ambulance service and Life Flight continued to arrive with increasingly strident reminders that payment was overdue. I contacted them all, more than once, to inform them I was on top of things and trying to get them paid. Nothing made them happy until I could call with a case file number and say he'd been approved for medical assistance. Really, I understand. Smaller businesses run much closer to the bone.

After a quick transfer between OHSU and the rehabilitation center, we were unprepared for the month-long wait to transfer Tracy from the rehabilitation center to the Rehabilitation Institute of Oregon (RIO). As time dragged on, I was in almost daily contact with representatives of both trying to determine why he was not being moved. All I could deduce, because no one wanted to say anything unprofessional, was that Oregon Health Plan staff was holding up things due to funding issues. It wasn't clear whether there was enough money to fund Tracy's transfer to RIO. Rehabilitation center staff assured me that they would be just as capable of guiding Tracy to his best possible recovery as RIO. It would just take them a bit longer. Obviously, the cost to the State was less at the rehabilitation center. I knew the staff meant well, but I wasn't sure it was more than wishful thinking. I also wanted the unique medical evaluations that RIO would offer.

Throughout the summer, I continued to get random questions from various representatives of the Oregon State Department of Human Services, Seniors and People with Disabilities "group." While I spoke with some representatives more than once, most often it was a new person each time. I discovered the art of asking for their own phone number before we finished talking so I had a fall-back position for later. They all had trouble understanding the self-employment income information for Tracy and repeatedly requested more information in a different format with a different due date. Inevitably, they wanted information faxed to them. I explained more than once that I was neither a caseworker nor did I have a fax machine. I lived in a private residence and I was the sister of a stroke victim for whom I cared deeply and was trying to help.

When I came to a blind corner in the bureaucratic world, I called Tracy's friend, Allan, the psychologist. He worked in another state but he worked for a similar bureaucracy and he understood the general rules. He was able to help me back out of blind corners and redirect my journey so I was productive instead of frustrated.

Those same representatives of various agencies also had great difficulty following Tracy's geographic movements. He had lived in Lincoln County, Oregon, was taken to OHSU which is in Multnomah County, and then to the rehabilitation center which is in Washington County. They couldn't decide where to "process" his application. I'm not sure the central computer ever got his address right, even months later. I telephoned a caseworker from Lincoln County, a great lady recommended by some of Tracy's friends who had worked with her in the past. Because she was very good at what she did, she was overwhelmed with cases. She explained that while she might eventually become Tracy's caseworker if/when he ever moved back to Lincoln City, currently we should work with the county where he was staying. At that point, it was Multnomah. So, after several more phone calls, I found the phone number for the Office Director in Multnomah County and talked with him. He explained the process of what occurs after an application for assistance is received; with whom I should get in contact; what the varying rules were depending on program and county; and very thoughtfully said I could feel free to contact him again. A hint to others who find themselves in a similar situation. Try to work with the caseworker/agent with whom you are first connected. Often you will need to work your way up the line. But if you take the time to start at the beginning, those along the way are more willing to help rather than re-route you back to the beginning. If you play by their rules, at least at the beginning, they appreciate it.

I cannot be appreciative enough of the Oregon Health Plan (OHP) and its payment on behalf of my brother to the hospitals, Life Flight, the ambulance, doctors, the rehabilitation center and for the purchase of prescriptions. Later after he came to live at our home, we, the patient/family and the OHP, no longer had apparent common purpose, and they and their surrogate, CareOregon, were not nearly so helpful. But OHP was there for the big early items and both OHP and CareOregon paid for Tracy's many and costly prescriptions. The Oregon Health Plan was Oregon's way of dealing with unfunded needs served by Medicaid. It was a precursor to the Affordable Care Act. I shudder to think of what might have happened to Tracy had Oregon not had this program in place.

In summary, I learned I was not alone, although many times I felt as though I was very much alone. Somebody had to take the lead. and I was that *somebody*. Early exhaustion and spent adrenalin helped me realize that I could not do everything by myself.

I took a giant leap into space knowing I needed two things: help when I asked (and I taught myself how to do that), and one regular afternoon off each week to rest and recharge, trusting that Tracy was in good hands even though I was not at his side.

I had to call upon all my capabilities and life experiences to move through each day and each week. I came to realize that I had reserves and strength previously unknown to me, and that I must use them all, leaving everything I had on the playing field. I also focused my anger at what had happened to Tracy, of which I had plenty, on accomplishing something that needed doing. Anger and fear for Tracy got me started but commitment to Tracy and support from my loved ones kept me going.

After our little family fell apart when my sister died, I took on the role of translator between my parents and surrogate mother to my new young brother, Tracy. I learned to put myself last. I recall one winter when I rode an early bus to school, I was supposed to have money for a school hot lunch. Mom wanted dad to give me the money; he didn't' have it, so I stood in their bedroom doorway waiting to see if it materialized. Usually it didn't and I had to run up the driveway from the house so I wouldn't miss the bus. In tense situations such as explaining to my mother who worked nights why dad couldn't come to the phone because he was "busy," which really meant he had locked the bathroom door and was drinking his dinner, I became adept at thinking up plausible scenarios. When my parents took a collective deep breath on their way to a real shouting match, I learned how to step in, deflect and explain to one what the other "really" meant. I also became a great weather forecaster. When it sounded like thunder was looming in the house, I whisked Tracy away and diverted his attention from what our parents were doing. I also learned to dissemble with teachers and principals who knew something was wrong. By age 12, I realized if a problem was to be solved, a situation bettered, and my life itself meaningful, I would have to do it all myself. I couldn't depend on anyone else. If I were dogged enough and worked hard enough, I believed I could make things turn out the way I wanted them to.

My brother had had a simple but full life complete with many friends. They knew more about his day-to-day life than I did. They wanted to help. We reached out to each other. I leaned on them. They gave so much. His friends became my friends.

At some point, I began to understand that this was not like a TV drama that would be over in an hour with all the loose ends neatly tied up. I shuddered as I realized that I couldn't see very far down the road I was on, much less see its end.

I learned who my own friends were, reached out to them, leaned on them. They carried me through. Without weekly bridge games with my "bridge sisters," I would have been consigned to an old-fashioned loony bin, and rightly so.

This life-changing event within our family strained the fabric that held us together in ways I hadn't expected. Everyone responds uniquely to a sudden and unpleasant event. Some reach out. Some deny the seriousness of the situation. Others retreat to what they know -- what's predictable in their lives – so they can once again find sound footing. Each is trying to find the best mode in which to survive and get through to the other side of a difficult situation.

There are experts out there: doctors, social workers, caseworkers, therapists, office managers, receptionists, paper shufflers, and they almost always know their stuff. I accepted that they have their rules, and I learned to deal with them. But, I also learned that I could lean on them and ask for help. If I asked the right question of the wrong person (the right church, wrong pew situation) I could also ask them where I should turn next. Almost all of them tried to help and many had good suggestions. If the person I was talking to couldn't/wouldn't help, I asked for the next person up the line. I learned not to leave the phone conversation or my place at the head of the line without having at least a hint of where to turn to next. I can think of just two entities that were unhelpful -- Tracy's credit union and the Internal Revenue Service (IRS).

Don't be afraid to go to the top: I called the Governor's Office. The person who took my call was a little surprised, but eventually I got a phone call back from the head of the agency in which I had become totally lost in a bureaucratic blur. The next time I contacted the local office of that agency, I used the Department head's name and I received quick assistance.

Finally, I figured mom had been right: Be Nice.

Part 2:
Back Out in the World,
But Not Quite …

Chapter 1:
Happy Birthday Tracy, October 6, 2011 …

We began yet another new routine. This one was being at home, but not at Tracy's home, until he was ready to really move home – back to Lincoln City. That time was so far in the future. I wondered, was that ever to be? We had to try. Tracy always had been so independent, and he needed his "alone" time. He would never feel he had moved on from this overwhelming "event" unless he could actually go home. Only by going home would he truly be able to take up his own life again.

On Tracy's birthday, I recalled other birthdays we had celebrated. A great one was in Eugene many years ago, where Bill and I and Tracy sat outside at Café Soriya enjoying the soft autumn evening. About 10 p.m., the fall rains began, softly at first, but then with certainty. We laughed about Tracy's birthday highlighting the change of season. We spent a more recent birthday with Tracy in Rome. Bill told him that he really knew how to party! That was another soft night where we sat out through the evening under the stars. And now, another milestone on Tracy's birthday: coming home, sort of.

The new "at-home" daily routine began with an ambitious plan of exercise, good meals and mental and physical stimulation. That was my idea. Reality soon reared its ugly head. No day lived up to the plan I had for it. Tracy was exhausted from his intense activity at the Rehabilitation Institute of Oregon. In the days that followed his coming home, it took all his energy to get up at the beginning of the day and get to the family room. He always was quiet in the morning, but since his stroke, fuzzy thinking, dizziness and nausea haunted his mornings. It would be enough to send me back to bed, and sometimes that's what happened to him.

I would open his bedroom door at 7:30 a.m. and he got to the family room after 9:00. At first, I listened and when I could tell he was stirring, I went into his room trying to judge when he'd need help getting into his wheel chair. First, he'd work to sit up, moving to the side of his bed. At the beginning, he'd sit there, motionless, head bent and eyes closed. I waited until he raised his head and looked at me. He always had a smile for me. Then, I helped him get his shirt on and after his morning bathroom break (for which I stood in the hall listening for the first week), I'd help him get dressed. Socks were well beyond his ability. Getting up at all was a challenge. He tipped over often and fell more than once, back onto his bed, on his way into the bathroom or leaning over the sink brushing his teeth. By the time he got out to his easy chair in the family room, he slid into it, closed his eyes, and was very quiet until I pestered him about breakfast (he didn't want any) and morning medications. He never had liked breakfast at breakfast time but the problem now was, he was supposed to take various medications with meals. He resisted because he was tired of vomiting. Who could blame him? I tried all sorts of food for breakfast (pizza anyone?). Even in tiny amounts. It was all a challenge.

Alison came over in the mornings with the intention of doing many creative exercises with Tracy: reading, speech, standing, math, identifying pictures. Therapists had drilled into us that the first six months were critical to Tracy's recovery. Progress was harder after that, they said. I wondered if we would all turn into pumpkins in six months, like Cinderella's carriage did at midnight. Alison found a great place called the Learning Palace that had terrific tools to use. The Learning Palace is a family-owned and locally operated store that provides educational materials and specialty toys to parents, teachers and homeschoolers. Husband-and-wife team Norman and Norma Faris opened the first Learning Palace in March of 1982 in Portland, Oregon. As a mom, Norma became frustrated with the lack of high-quality educational products available for her four children. She suggested to her husband that they open a teaching supply store. Today, they offer their products in five local stores and online.

While the Learning Palace is primarily for helping young people, after Alison talked with them about what she was trying to do with Tracy, they were very interested and helpful. It seems to me that we will have more need for places like the Learning Palace to provide primary educational exercises made for adults who have suffered traumatic brain injury. It's a delicate issue: the necessary tools for speech and reading, for example, are identical for both children and injured adults, but adults are not children.

The RIO therapists had given us some exercises, printed on paper, to use with Tracy until we could see his new therapists who would treat him as an out-patient. All the exercises Alison tried took a toll on Tracy. We dialed it 'way back. He couldn't focus on what was on TV. He didn't want to wear his glasses. He was immediately nauseated by trying to read. His eyes couldn't scan the width of a page without fluttering. When asked to identify animals with names that began with an "L", he couldn't think of any. But when we asked him to name animals from Africa, he thought of two. When asked to look at any picture to identify anything in it, he vomited. We tried showing him pictures of anything outdoors because he loved the outdoors. He'd try. Then he'd close his eyes and sit totally still. Sometimes that worked. At first, mostly it didn't. He'd throw-up.

Tracy needed to rest after each separate activity: getting up, getting through morning washing face/brushing teeth/combing hair routine, getting dressed, getting to the family room, eating whatever breakfast we could convince him to eat, and perhaps a visit from a friend and maybe an exercise or two with Alison. While Alison visited with Tracy, I made his lunch. He liked lunch and we used it as a reward for a productive morning and as a way for him to begin to tell time during the day. When I asked him what time it was, he didn't say "noon or 12:30," he said, "Lunch time!" After lunch, Tracy took a short stint in his easy chair, then he wheeled down the hall for a two-plus hour nap in his quiet room. After napping, he'd repeat his pattern of getting up slowly and carefully, return to the family room and sit quietly, sometimes just sitting or sometimes "watching TV" with his eyes closed. When it wasn't raining outside, one of us would wheel him out and around the driveway and the sidewalk just so he had some fresh air. Later in the afternoon, I'd talk at him as I was making dinner. It was my time to help him formulate ideas and to express his opinion as to how the day had gone. At various times Alison and I would ask him to journal, but it was always a monumental task for him. After dinner, I'd invite him to read, or be read to, or look at any pictures. He'd decline and then we'd "watch TV." I would use that time to get the next day organized. He'd take his "night" medication, and go to bed around 9:30 p.m., sleeping ten to eleven hours at first. I flopped into bed right after because I was exhausted, too, although I'm sure in a very different way.

Being focused on Tracy's needs while he was under the direct care of hospital or rehab center staff worked very differently than when he was at home. In addition to direct care for Tracy, many other important activities required attention like paying bills and keeping track of his paintings, arranging and transporting him to doctor and lab visits, getting therapy approved for him, and filling out lots and lots of new paperwork. I truly began to appreciate all the work that had been performed on his behalf while he was in some form of institutionalized care. Gone were the skilled-care nurses and medical assistants and people who made meals and changed beds. I had help from family and friends at home and I delegated to them when I could, but I was definitely on my own. As a caregiver, once I set my course, it was hard to switch gears and think of something that someone else could do to help. It took more energy to think up something, describe it and delegate it than it was worth. That's what happens to caregivers. Ultimately, they are on their own.

At first, Tracy got his physical exercise wheeling up-and-down the hallway in our home and by transferring from wheelchair to bed/bath/chair. Standing up to brush his teeth was exhausting. Six weeks after he came home, he began to use the walker up-and-down the hallway with Bill close behind; and then, a couple of months after that, he started walking a few steps unaided before he fell sideways; then he managed the thirteen steps up-and-down the hall on his own, again with Bill close behind. It was a great day when he walked the entire length of the hallway in one uninterrupted try.

Representatives of CareOregon and the Oregon Health Plan were not helpful when it came to the provision of a wheel chair, the purchase of other needed items such as a shower bench, a special toilet seat, installation of a ramp at the front door so he could enter and leave the house, and rehabilitation therapy supplies. When asked for assistance to help pay for the wheel chair, they indicated that a wheel chair was necessary purely to get him into and around the inside of our house. Since we already had that one, for which WE had paid the first month's rent and for which they would not reimburse us, the response was, "Nonetheless..." They didn't care about his ability to travel outside the house and that also went for the wheel chair ramp on the front porch. As far as they were concerned, it was not necessary because he was already in the house. They didn't really care about whether he ever got out again. When I asked how we were supposed to take him to appointments for doctors and therapy, they said for medically necessary purposes, they would pay for van transport – the same van transport that the occupational therapist at the rehabilitation center said she didn't want Tracy to use because the rocking of wheel chairs in the van as it traveled down the road would make him very sick. When I pointed that out, I was told again that there was van transport available and if he had to get to a hospital we always could call an ambulance. At that point, I gave up trying to get their help.

Rather than renting a generic wheel chair which didn't "fit" him, we wanted to purchase one tailored to his physical needs. The current rented wheel chair didn't fit him well and, therefore, was uncomfortable. It was also very heavy. We had no idea how long he would need a wheel chair, but believed it would certainly be more than a month or two. First, I checked Craig's List for a used lighter weight wheel chair. I soon discovered that while there were many wheel chairs on the list, most of them were smaller: used chairs that come available often are a child's chair, which the child has outgrown. Other available chairs were motorized and for people larger than Tracy. So, I sought input from friends, dug into the internet, found a light-weight wheel chair offered by a local provider named United Seating and Mobility, loaded Tracy into my car without his current clunky wheel chair, took him to a warehouse area south of town, and got him "fitted" for a wheel chair and custom seat. We brought the wheel chair home and the seat followed several days later. The seat was more important than I realized: anyone trying to use either a generic wheel chair or someone else's chair struggles with fit; circulation to the legs is often impaired while back and shoulder problems also are common. The seat itself cost more than $200. It was worth every penny for Tracy's comfort. Another reason to get the wheel chair "fitted," was to be sure it was sized for him. Both the height and the depth of the seat should be tailored to the user. Relatives and friends paid for his wheel chair and the other "enrichments" needed to make his life easier. I love the word "enrichments," that's truly what members of the medical-equipment community call them. It's a nice word but a little odd in its application, I think. Tracy needed and used that wheel chair for many months. Slowly its use lessened to those situations requiring a long walk or long periods of standing. The day came, more than a year later, when we put it out in the garage and then, finally, into the upstairs attic – close enough at hand but out of sight.

Previously very fastidious, Tracy did not want to take showers. He hated them because they made him so cold. We agreed that he needed at least one a week. (More than a year later, he got back to his former routine of a shower each morning.) On shower day, I'd warm the bathtub and get the shower warm. I'd keep the door closed to get the room warm. I'd get all his clothes in there so he could dress where it was warmest. For the first few months, I helped him transfer to the shower bench because he couldn't do it alone. We got baby shampoo because the others stung his eyes and he couldn't keep them shut tight enough to keep the soap out. I'd hold the towel over the heat register along with his terrycloth bathrobe to try to capture all the warmth I could. When the warm water was turned off, he started shivering so hard I was concerned he'd fall off the shower bench. I became adept at getting the towel around him fast followed just as quickly by the bathrobe.

After a summer of not cooking and doing the wash for anyone, I was again doing those chores full-time. Usually, Bill made his own dinner. While we often ate together, Bill and I had eaten separate meals for years since we liked different foods. We'd invite each other to dinner once in awhile and cook for each other. Sometimes we'd go out to dinner. It all worked out. Now I was cooking for Tracy and me and since I am what my family calls a "Rabbit Food Eater," and he is not, I was preparing two different meals at a time.

Luckily, Bill didn't mind shopping. I prepared menus and grocery lists to last a week, and he went and got the food I needed. After consulting with Tracy's doctors, I was trying very hard to cook him the kinds of meals they said he should eat to gain weight and get healthy. Some of that was not what he wanted to eat. Green leafy vegetables were beyond his ability to swallow for many months. He hated vinegar, thus almost all salad dressings. Vegetables smelled bad to him. He continued to have problems with swallowing and nausea. His left hand was weak; his right hand almost uncontrollable, so eating was a challenge. I had his meal ready to eat when I put the plate in front of him because I didn't want to cut up his food while he watched. His sensory taste and smell receptors were still off. If I cooked an egg whether he was in the room or not, he could smell it and it revolted him.

We were lucky in that Tracy was able to take care of himself toilet-wise. To keep from getting up in the middle of the night – which is problematic for someone as dizzy as he was – he used a urinal. To keep his bed fresh, I found it necessary to change his sheets and pillow cases often because he sweat so heavily when he slept. Somewhere along the way, before he came to live with us, he developed a fungus on the skin of his back, which required attention every day, and his feet continued to need a regular slathering of lotion because they were so dry. I learned that skin is considered a major organ and Tracy's was struggling. He never, as far as I knew, had skin issues before. I put out clean shirts, underwear and socks daily to keep his skin as clean as possible. I was washing and drying clothes, sheets, and towels more frequently than before.

I structured my day to be close at hand when Tracy was awake. His most "dangerous" times were when he got up-or-down, in-or-out of a chair or bed, and when he went into the bathroom. Falling and the possibility of his hitting his head created nightmares for me. I jumped awake in a fright more than once, listening to determine whether I'd actually heard him fall. As days went by, I looked out at my garden that had gone on without me all summer. Now in the fall, it was time to put it to bed and turn the compost piles. I had little time to do all that all at once, but found I could be very productive in the couple of hours Tracy was down for his afternoon nap. Besides, by that time of day, if I sat down, I'd fall asleep. It was much better to go outside. My friends Mary and Karla came over to help with moving plants around in the front garden. Gardens are never finished. I was eyeing the front garden all summer as I went about my day, deciding what I would prefer over what was there. They came and helped make it happen.

Early Saturday mornings became the time I sorted Tracy's medications for the week. At first, he was taking twelve medications and they needed to be sorted by when he took them. Some also needed to be cut in half. I found whacking a serrated table knife with the hard back of the small brush (the one that I used to brush the cat) under a kitchen towel to keep pieces of pills from flying all over did the trick. It was cheaper than paying the pharmacy to split the pills in half. The Oregon Health Plan paid for Tracy's medications, for which I am very grateful. However, they wouldn't pay for some dosages or splitting pills, hence the need to get the higher dosage and cut it in half myself.

Tracy never had been diabetic, but one of his body's many difficulties as a result of his stroke was that his blood sugar shot up and his pancreas appeared to be struggling to work. In fact, all his major organs were struggling to right themselves. Once in the morning and once at night, over time and with lots of practice, I became adept at pricking his finger, putting a sample of his blood on a small tape, inserting it into a meter, and recording the results. At first it was horribly difficult. I hated making him wince and jump when I pricked his finger. We took and recorded his blood pressure several times throughout the day, but always first thing in the morning. Although I don't know this for a fact, I would bet Tracy rarely, if ever, took his blood pressure prior to his stroke. He was more attuned to things like heart rate and proper breathing when he exercised. Now we faithfully kept a journal that also included any unexpected happenings: not feeling well, being physically and/or mentally slower than usual, falling down, vomiting, etc. At first, I recorded it all. Later, Tracy took on the job, laboriously writing blood-pressure numbers, pulse rate and other notes.

I had given up the last of my volunteer work and something was always interrupting the nightly news on TV, so I discovered early morning news programs just to keep me in touch with the rest of the world. The only quiet time I had for months was in the early morning. I jealously protected that time. And, my weekly bridge games with my Bridge Sisters were heaven-sent.

During the mornings when Alison was with Tracy, I visited with various other people on the phone: doctors' offices, the pharmacy, the administrative office for the rehabilitation therapists, representatives of CareOregon and the Oregon Health Plan, and the Department of Human Services/Seniors and People with Disabilities, student loans, Social Security and Supplemental Security Income (SSI), Tracy's credit union and their collection agency, credit card companies, art-gallery owners, accountants about taxes, and even an attorney about the possibility of declaring bankruptcy for Tracy.

A good example of how a simple job can eat time and become overly complex was the pharmacy situation. The doctors at RIO had written the prescriptions Tracy needed for a month after he moved to our house. The plan was that we would refill his prescriptions once a month. We stopped by the pharmacy on the way home from RIO to pick them up. Some were not available at that pharmacy, and the Oregon Health Plan (OHP) had not yet authorized any of them. We began a close and personal relationship with two outstanding Rite Aid pharmacists. They were very helpful in the almost two years we dealt with them about Tracy's medications. They re-contacted OHP and got the authorization straightened out. Bill went back the next day to pick up the medications. Over time, the 30-day supply/pickup plan fell apart. Some medications were changed by the doctors part-way through a cycle and some were subsequently switched back, or dosages were modified, or a different generic was ordered. The upshot was that we were picking up prescriptions once or twice a week, not once a month. The reason I was cutting pills in half was that the doctors reduced dosages, but OHP didn't pay for the smaller dosage, so we kept getting the bigger doses, but cut the pill in half. That also meant that we had more pills, and when I sought to get the amount cut back because we were using half as many, we found that OHP couldn't supply less than 30 days at a time. Periodically, we took all the unused pills to the Police Department for disposal. If Tracy lived alone, I have no idea how he would have coped with his medications.

We decided Tracy should carry a basic telephone just for emergencies. Bill picked one up and we added Tracy to our plan. We programmed our own phone numbers into his Speed Dial and made sure he knew how to use it to call us or 911. He was very good about carrying that phone with him. That way, I felt more comfortable when I went outside to the garden during his afternoon naps. I always carried my own phone so he could call me if he was in distress. Of course if he fell before he called, that negated the plan and I worried about that, too. About the same time, Bill picked up some fuzzy slippers for Tracy. They needed to have traction so he could use his feet to propel the wheelchair, but they also needed to be warm. He had running and walking shoes, but his feet needed additional shoes to keep them healthy. I checked his feet, toes and toenails daily. I rubbed them with lotion daily. That helped with circulation and I could see right away if there were any problems. Somewhere along the line, one of Tracy's big toenails had been injured. It was growing oddly and needed to be clipped with care so it didn't become ingrown. After having a doctor treat it once, I made sure Tracy got regular pedicures so his nails were taken care of.

The ladies at Elegant Nails were so very sweet. The first time Tracy met them, they looked at him and told him to stay in his wheelchair, and one lady knelt on a pillow on the floor to cut his toenails. He couldn't get into their fancy chair with the footbath and extensive menu of back massages. The smell of nail polish remover made him very queasy, so they moved his chair right by the front door with the door open to get fresh air and worked on his toes there. It was late fall and cold, but no one complained. Later, when he did make it into the chair, the motion of the back massage made him vomit. (At that point, we discovered one of the ladies had a real aversion to that act and she joined him.) As time progressed, they cheered him when he came into the shop because each time he was doing so much better. Even now I get pedicures there and the ladies always ask after Tracy. He loved getting his toes painted outrageous colors: black, dark purple, silver and wild bright lime green. A note about the need for pedicures: For several months, Tracy was relegated to a wheelchair and he also was being treated for diabetes. Both cause significant circulatory issues that affect the lower extremities and Tracy couldn't care for his own feet. He couldn't focus well enough to see them and neither hand worked well. I have arthritis in my hands and fingers and so am unable to clip his nails properly. I can't stress how important pedicures are for continued foot health of someone like Tracy.

A few days after Tracy came "home," I took a good look at him. He looked scary. His hair hadn't been cut for months, his eyebrows had decided to grow a lot, and the hair in his ears was unreal. This was pretty much all new. I called his nephew, my son, and asked when he and his son, Trenton, were going for their manly grooming. It happened to be coming up on the next Saturday. We made arrangements to meet them at the hairdresser's. Denise was sweet with Tracy. She cut his hair with fingers that barely touched him because his head and neck were supersensitive to touch. She also didn't insist on washing his hair first since leaning his head back onto a hard sink edge to wash his hair would not be good. She trimmed, edged and fluffed, and made him a "new" man. He enjoyed the give-and-take between her, Mitch and Trenton. His hair didn't grow as fast as it used to. Later, Tracy would come with me when I got my hair cut and darling Laure would cut both of us for the price of my cut. She was always gentle with Tracy and as he progressed over time, they had conversations and laughs while he was in her chair. To this day, she keeps up with Tracy via Facebook.

Bill returned from a trip the night before Tracy came to live with us and he was home for a few days before he left again. Earlier, he had gotten tickets to the ballet and a play over the weekend. Again, he was celebrating "getting our lives back" by starting the cultural season with a bang. Alison came to stay with Tracy while Bill and I went out. I tried not to fall asleep during the performances. Dinner was fun, though.

In October and November, the number of visitors slowed. In the early days when we were all so scared for Tracy, and when they needed to see him to reassure themselves that he was still on this Earth, they came almost every day. Later, when he needed them again, they were there once more.

Those who visited brought thoughtful gifts: blankets and sweaters to keep him warm, get-well charms like a ceramic fish, massages, tasty tidbits of food to entice him to eat, and sometimes just plain warm conversation bringing him news of his friends and his home at the ocean. They would rearrange the chairs and stools and cushions so they sat in front of Tracy and either equal with or below his line of sight. It was helpful to keep his eyes from roving across his field of vision, which would trigger nausea. When groups of friends visited, I would ask Tracy to try to focus on one person rather than scanning the group. They all reminded him to look at one person at a time, laughing that no one would be offended if he didn't look at them right away.

Tracy always loved a wide variety of music. Many of Tracy's friends are musicians. Evans and his girlfriend, Anita, came to visit one day. Evans is a well-traveled world-class musician now living up the Siletz River south of Lincoln City. His house is on the "wrong" side of the highway, which means anyone visiting the house parks on the road-side of the river and takes a little boat with a set of rope pulleys from one ramp to another by the house, across the river. Evans has a grand piano, which came to the house via barge. Tracy lived at Evans' house for a time, sleeping on the second floor with his kayak hung outside the bedroom window and noting that cows in the field surrounding Evans' house were a good gauge of how high the river was: the higher the river, the closer to the house the cows came. Once, when the river flooded, the Coast Guard helicopter flew over and they offered to hoist Evans to safety. Since the offer didn't include his dog, Evans didn't go.

When he visited Tracy, Evans brought a lightweight cardboard instrument for Tracy to play. He also brought new, soft strings for Tracy's guitar – to be ready when Tracy wanted to play it again. Evans had taught Tracy on the guitar in the past, and we hoped trying to finger the chords might help him return to the music he loved. Up to this point, Tracy had politely but adamantly refused to listen to music because it caused confusion in his head. He also couldn't make either hand work the way he wanted.

Kelly, Tracy's glass-artist friend, and her kids visited one day bringing brightly colored tissue paper, card stock, colored felt-tip pens, snub-nosed scissors and glue. They sat with Tracy at the kitchen table making all sorts of cards. At first, Tracy just wanted to sit there and watch, but the kids enticed him into drawing lines and designing the cut-up tissue paper on the card stock and then getting into the glue. Laughter rang around the room before they finished.

During this period of Alison's life, there was good news and bad news. The good news was mostly for Tracy and me because she was able to spend days and days with us. She was not working. The bad news was for her: she had injured her shoulder on the job, was in substantial chronic pain due to the injury, and her employer was balking at paying for any medical treatment. She went to her doctor who wouldn't treat her for an on-the-job injury. She tried to work, but even though her doctor told the company that she couldn't extend her arm and lift anything weighing more than ten pounds without incurring further injury, they kept putting her in situations where that was exactly what they wanted her to do. Unfortunately, her employer is one of those big companies that can "self-insure" themselves. In my opinion, the company had almost complete autonomy and the State exercised very little authority. They ran her around unmercifully for second and third medical opinions and competing and incomprehensible paperwork. The company even cancelled a scheduled surgery the night before it was to take place. The one good thing she got was a few physical-therapy visits (which they later tried to charge her for). Because she couldn't drive, I drove her to doctor's appointments and to some meetings either the company or the State required. When you injure your right shoulder, it's impossible to shift gears on a car. The forward motion is excruciating. If I didn't drive her, other friends did. Alison was in limbo for months.

The bright time of her day was being with Tracy. Tracy always had been her protector even when she was little. Later, when they lived together while both attended the University of Oregon, Alison more than once got herself into situations that snowballed downhill fast. Tracy always was there for her. Now she was able to do something to help him, and she did. Alison is humorous. She made up stories about words she wanted Tracy to remember. She'd put together animals and places and ask if he could connect them, in some instances, complete with cartoon pictures. She read to him. She did a lot of "Remember when we…" stories about trips we had taken together. Alison had Tracy complete fill-in-the-blank exercises we had gotten from the Rehabilitation Institute of Oregon (RIO). One thing we noticed was that speed had to be removed from the equation. If put under pressure to perform "as quickly as possible," Tracy became totally flustered, frustrated and was no longer willing to participate in the exercise.

Sometimes Bill took Tracy for walks, but often it was Alison who did this. In the beginning, the "walk" was in the wheel chair out to the driveway and back. Later, with the walker, Bill followed directly behind Tracy. He said he watched which way Tracy started leaning and so got a head start on which direction he started to fall. Bill also noticed that while the walker's front wheels worked fine on the sidewalk, the back legs dragged and skidded. He found some little plastic skis and attached them to the rear legs. The walker worked much more smoothly after that. When Alison walked with Tracy, she got him to the driveway, where she had put out the orange Gelato Cones (brought by Joel and Liz to the rehabilitation center the summer before). She laid them out so he serpentined around them. The single way he could turn was by taking little baby steps, stopping between each one. No matter how cold it was, the effort of turning was so great that beads of sweat broke out on his forehead. He could turn right better than left. Using the Gelato Cones was a real challenge for him, but he kept at it. Every day that it wasn't pouring rain or too cold, one of us had him outside walking and navigating around the cones.

And so, Tracy's first few months "at home" settled into a routine for us that included pretty full days: pedicures, watching football games on TV, taking the kitties to the vet for their annual checkups, celebration of my son's fiftieth birthday, bridge for me, and rounds of doctor's appointments and physical therapy – not all for Tracy, but also for Alison, with her injured shoulder.

Each day was a new beginning. The daily adventure was that we didn't know how Tracy would feel when he awoke in the morning. We came to realize we couldn't assume that this morning would pick up where he left off yesterday. Sometimes it did, but often in the beginning of his days at our house, he regressed. On bad days, he was more curled into himself, quiet, not hungry or thirsty. They were often the days with more than usual difficulties with balance and nausea. Trying to coax him to drink anything was a chore – more for him than for me. He continued to choke on any thin liquid, like water. We had instructions to follow from speech therapists he had seen at the rehabilitation center and RIO, but in the beginning, he was unable to remember the exercises or the instructions. We'd go over them. He knew he was supposed to know what to do, but he couldn't remember and it frustrated him. Early on he would ball up his hands into fists and hit his forehead. We stopped him from doing that, telling him how dangerous it was for him. He then would take a breath, close his eyes and when he re-opened them, he would have regained control. I realized I couldn't leave home a lot and never be away for long. Tracy had great judgment but lousy balance so there were endless possibilities of "what if he falls and someone is not right there?"

Chapter 2:
Coming Back:
Computer Games, Silos and Whirling Tops

In mid-October, 2011, I took Tracy to his first round of rehabilitation therapies as an outpatient. That was with a Legacy occupational therapist eleven days after his last therapy sessions at RIO, followed two days later with appointments for physical therapy and speech therapy. Those appointments were south of us, down the I-5 freeway. On the day in between, he first saw his new doctor at the Legacy Good Samaritan Physicians Clinic near downtown Portland. Just like Doernbecher Children's Hospital earlier, Good Samaritan Hospital brought back sad memories for me. Sherry, my deceased sister, also had spent time at Good Sam. I hadn't been back in the area until I took Tracy to the clinic. Parts of it looked the same after more than 60 years. The first time we went into Portland to Good Sam, I drove via the freeway and discovered that our exit was closed for the day. After getting almost to the Washington State border before I could find a way to turn around, I decided to come up with an alternate route. From then on, I drove the Barnes Road/Burnside surface streets route and found it much prettier and less hectic.

We came to really like the doctors at the Physicians Clinic. Their clientele was an interesting mix of "regular" people and people who lived on the street. The doctors without exception were terrific. Most were young; but a few were older, acting as great mentors. The doctors were very willing to work with us to try to reduce the quantity of medication Tracy was taking. They spent time with Tracy, talking with him directly. Both of us appreciated that. As time went on, people who dealt with Tracy realized that while he spoke with difficulty, his brain was reawakening. It took time, but when people took the time, they could have a decent conversation with him.

As to his continuing rehabilitation, I found that obtaining therapeutic treatment as an outpatient was totally different from that provided while he was hospitalized or living in a rehabilitation/care center. The difference was - - *insurance*. When Tracy was at RIO, he was prescribed a long-term treatment plan which was to bridge relatively seamlessly from the facility to his living at home. Once Tracy left RIO, he was transferred to CareOregon, an organization that acted as the administrator for the Oregon Health Plan in our geographic area and covered home treatment for individuals. Under CareOregon, we selected a doctor and various medical-service groups from the CareOregon list of approved providers. OHP paid for the treatment he received at RIO, which is a Legacy facility.

When we contacted the outpatient therapy facilities at Legacy, we were told Tracy's first visit would be to evaluate his current condition and prospective ability to improve, even though they had access to all of RIO's reports regarding work that had already been completed there. The insurance provider required the additional evaluation. After that, a treatment plan would be written and sent to CareOregon and the Oregon Health Plan for approval. Maybe CareOregon and the Oregon Health Plan weren't surprised, but none of the non-bureaucrats expected it to take as long as it did.

Tracy waited for six weeks for his next therapy appointment: December 1, 2011 with Daria, the terrific speech therapist. I had called Legacy and CareOregon at least once a week to determine what was holding things up. They kept saying "soon." During one of the phone calls to CareOregon, I was told that after six months (from the date of Tracy's stroke) his condition would be considered "chronic" and therefore he would no longer be eligible for any therapy – I could feel their shrug over the phone. What would be the use, he was as good as he was going to be. On dark days, I began to wonder if they were deliberately waiting for the six-month "drop dead" date so they didn't' have to pay for additional therapy. That would be one way to weed out people from an already overburdened and under-funded medical system.

When we saw Daria in December, she said her first and second proposed treatment plans were sent back by CareOregon/Oregon Health Plan. For all three therapies (physical, occupational, and speech) there had been requirements for reapplication, pre-approval, assessment, submission of a "plan" for each therapy, minor adjustments and requests for resubmission. All this took up the limited time before the Oregon Health Plan would no longer pay for therapy. Some applications were resubmitted because initial applications were misplaced. We had such a limited amount of time to get help -- only until the last of December. While we never received approval for any occupational therapy and approval for just one physical therapy visit for a specific vestibular (balance) evaluation, before the December deadline, all of a sudden, there was approval for so many speech-therapy appointments we couldn't get them all in before the end-of-the-year deadline. We managed to squeeze in seven appointments in three weeks even through the Christmas holidays.

On our first appointment with Daria, she met us in the waiting room and we stopped at the drinking fountain on the way to her office. She had tiny paper cups in her hand. She filled one and handed it to Tracy. He looked at it. She gave the others to Alison and me and invited us to fill them and come along. We did. I also carried Tracy's cup so it wouldn't spill as Alison pushed his wheelchair. In her office, she asked Tracy to drink the water. He said he wasn't very thirsty. She sweetly insisted. At that point, we all wondered, frankly, what the big deal was with the water. She was a SPEECH Therapist, not a water or drinking therapist, and we were in the mode of "get as much as possible out of this visit because there probably won't be any more." We didn't want to waste time doing a dance to get Tracy to drink a cup of water he didn't want.

Then Daria explained. Swallowing and speech go together. She would be working just as hard to help Tracy swallow properly as she would to help him regain his speech faculties. She tried many permutations to help Tracy drink: she cut out a tiny scallop on the cup's rim; she offered different sized straws; she even had him try drinking from the back of the cup. She dragged out an assortment of very interesting and complex pictures of the throat showing how it decides whether it's handling air or liquid and that nothing good happens when they get mixed up. Daria suggested ways for Tracy to practice a new way of swallowing. She said the part of his brain that ran this automatically had been damaged, particularly the part that finished closing off his throat to keep liquid from going to his lungs.

Daria elicited information from Tracy and was delighted to learn that he was a photographer and a painter and that he loved going to Hawaii. She loved Hawaii, too, and so they had something in common to use as they traveled on their Speech Path. She tried valiantly to interest him in playing the ukelele, but that never happened.

All-too-soon the session was over, but the delight was that for the remainder of the month, Tracy, Alison and I went every Tuesday and Thursday morning to see Daria. In one of those early meetings, Daria attempted to get Tracy engaged in conversation. Three of us -- Alison, Daria, and I -- couldn't recall the name of a famous drawing of a man by Leonardo da Vinci, finally giving up and moving on. After we returned home, Tracy had lunch and took his nap. When he got up, he took a yellow Post-It note along with a pencil to the table, and seemed very intent on doing something with them. I was working on dinner. Several minutes later, he motioned to me to take the Post-It note. On it he had laboriously lettered "Vitruvian Man." He was right; that was the name none of us could recall earlier in the day. As I recollected the conversation in Daria's office earlier that day, we had moved on, excluding Tracy from our deliberations. But he'd participated anyway – and got the last word.

Just before Christmas we got word that one more physical-therapy visit was approved, specifically to evaluate whether Tracy would benefit from vestibular (balance) therapy. This appointment was scheduled for the hour after one of Tracy's speech therapy visits. After Tracy, Alison and I got to the appointment, Emmy, the physical therapist, put him through his paces. As a result of Emmy's requests to show her how he was doing, Tracy fell over onto tumbling mats and into parallel bars, and the wall, and the drinking fountain, but she persisted. So did he. After the session, Emmy stated that she firmly believed vestibular therapy would be very beneficial for Tracy. She put together a treatment plan and submitted it for approval. All we heard was "No." So, we never saw Emmy again.

However, before we left our single appointment with Emmy, I asked if she could give us some exercises we could do at home. She did and I am so appreciative because we worked them to death and that was OK because we knew we were going in the right direction.

The exercises were interesting. For example, either Alison or I had Tracy stand in one corner of the kitchen/family room and face diagonally across the room to the other corner. Actually, at first, it was more that we leaned him kind of like a log against the wall in the corner. He couldn't stand up by himself, and he couldn't stand "naturally," rather he stood stiffly and awkwardly. Eventually, he could stand alone in the corner, looking out at the room. Then one of us would ask him to close his eyes and see how long he could stand there. At first, he tipped over immediately. (We stood in front of him and caught him before he went over.) We then put a brightly colored stuffed animal on the cats' tall play structure in the other corner of the room. We'd ask him to look at it with one eye, then the other, then both. When he started, he couldn't complete the exercise without falling over. He had difficulty focusing on something that far away.

In another exercise, Alison taped a small bright green rubber ball to the eraser portion of a pencil and moved it carefully across Tracy's field of vision. She asked him to follow it with his eyes. At first he moved his head to follow the ball and he could do the exercise just once before he was nauseated. It was many months before his eyes, especially his left eye, didn't flutter when he tried to look up and out.

Toward the end of November, 2011, Tracy received Notice of Action letters from CareOregon that stated "...Based on your age, for your chronic condition, your therapy benefit is 12 total visits per year. With the 12 visits approved, you have used up your benefits until 11/27/2012." That total, I think, included four original evaluation visits plus all the speech therapy visits that we could not get done within the time limit.

After the first of the year (January 2012) all of Tracy's applications for treatment were turned down. Until.... I read and re-read the multi-page Notice of Action denial forms from CareOregon and found something buried in the fourth paragraph that worked for us. "...However, Oregon Health Plan benefits do provide up to four (4) therapy re-evaluations in a 12-month period for your condition. Re-evaluations do not require preauthorization and should be used for periodic review and updating of your home treatment program." We began requesting re-evaluations every three months. When we met with the therapists, we asked for "homework" that would last about three months.

During this time, we also were notified that CareOregon/Oregon Health Plan were reducing dental benefits to non-pregnant recipients over the age of 21. We searched for a dentist who was a service provider under CareOregon, made an appointment and got Tracy in for a cleaning, exam and an appointment to pull a broken tooth before the benefits went away. This episode reinforced that caregivers may be the only line of defense for someone like Tracy. I hadn't thought to look into his mouth to be sure that everything was O.K.. Obviously, it wasn't. We had to get all this done before year's end when the benefits changed. In previous years, Tracy had taken good care of his teeth. But, that did not include many visits to a dentist because he couldn't afford it. After the benefits changed at the first of the year, from what I could deduce, cleaning would be paid for every three years.

We also received notification that food stamp (Supplemental Nutrition Assistance Program aka SNAP) benefits would be reduced as well. That didn't matter too much to us because we already had been told that we would have to do a major reconstruction of our kitchen (separate locked cabinets, a separate and identifiable section of the refrigerator, for example) to show an inspector who could come by with little notice that Bill and I were not stealing food from Tracy or misusing food stamps. I reminded the folks at the "Seniors and People with Disabilities" office that Tracy was joining us at our house; we were not living at his house. Didn't matter, so we declined to pursue food stamps for him. Trying to receive food stamps always would be a pain, we discovered, and the tiny amount they later decided Tracy could have was actually an insult. When I asked if the official telling me the amount Tracy "qualified" for had the same budget as Tracy did, there was silence on the other end of the phone. In fairness, I wouldn't want her job. Obviously, getting food stamps in this country is anything but a Snap.

Bill continued "social directing" with plays, symphonies and ballets for us to attend. Tracy and I joined him for a celebration of Veterans' Day at a local restaurant. It was raining and dark when we arrived and there were many others arriving at the same time. I noted many walkers, wheel chairs, canes, and people being leaned on. In a perverse way, I felt relief. This was a crowd in which Tracy wouldn't be misunderstood or cut in front of or stared at. Tracy handled the noise and hubbub well, but was very tired when he got home.

Sometime later, we took him to his first movie in months. We discovered the handicapped seating area in the theatre and sat next to Tracy, who was in his wheel chair, during the matinee. In each instance, we asked him first if he would like to go. I think he was torn: part of him wanted to stay home and not move, but the other part wanted to do anything that could help him get better. Usually, that part won.

Just as we had gotten settled into a routine, Tracy made life more "interesting." About three weeks after he arrived in Beaverton, he passed out and fell, or he fell and passed out. We were never sure because it happened after his afternoon nap as he was getting up. He was trying very hard to be as independent as possible, so he was trying to get up without help. He told me later that he followed all the rules, like sitting for awhile on the side of the bed with his legs dangling over before he stood up, and turned to get himself into the wheelchair which sat locked and ready for him next to the bed. But sometimes, the dizziness was so great, he just blacked out. This apparently was one of those times. When it was time for him to get up from his nap, I always opened his door and then listened for movement. On this occasion, I was not home. I was out playing bridge on my Monday afternoon off.

Bill didn't tell me what happened until that evening. (Again, the guilt just engulfed me because I positively and again unreasonably knew it wouldn't have happened had I been home.) Bill said it was no big thing, after he heard Tracy fall (the door was still closed), he helped get Tracy right side up and he said everything was fine. I asked if he had hit his head. Bill didn't know but Tracy said he had. I deduced he'd hit the side of his head, not the back. Both of them kept insisting Tracy was fine. As before, anger at Bill washed over me because he was not apparently concerned about what had happened and he didn't respond the way I would have.

The next day, Tracy had an early morning dental appointment and after I got him back home, I called his doctor at Physicians Clinic because Tracy seemed to me to be a little slower than usual. It could have been my imagination. It might have been caused by the local anesthetic he received during his visit to the dentist, but I wasn't sure. The result of my phone call was that I drove Tracy into Portland to Good Samaritan Hospital for a CT Scan the next morning. The doctor showed his concern, being very attentive to Tracy's behavior and speech. In order to request the Scan, Tracy had to sign something called an "Advance Beneficiary Notice of Noncoverage (ABN)" that said the scan was not covered for his condition and the cost (approximately $1,078.00) might not be paid by insurance. I thought, wow, this makes you feel good going into a scary procedure! I decided the need for the scan outweighed the potential fight regarding payment and told him he should do it. No one appeared upset that his signature was not at all like his previous signatures. But then, they hadn't ever seen his earlier signature. It turned out well: the procedure wasn't scary and the bill was paid, but it was an unsettling exerience.

Challenge and uncertainty continued as to how Tracy would feel each day. Every day was a brand new adventure. Sometimes, he would go to bed feeling pretty good, seemingly more aware of the world around him, and having been more involved in the general conversation. The next morning would be either good or bad and how he had felt the night before was totally irrelevant. Luckily, he never suffered the substantial physical pain that many stroke victims do. For that I am fervently grateful.

For some time I had wondered how much Tracy's lack of mental sharpness was the result of his stroke, and how much was the result of side effects to the many drugs he was taking. For example, he was taking a regular dose of an anti-nausea medicine, yet he was still throwing up. Was the medicine not working? Or, would it have been even worse without it? His doctors understood my concerns and talked with Tracy about what he thought. He said that he'd like to take fewer drugs with lesser dosages. On the other hand, the doctors were very cognizant of Tracy's medical condition: fluctuating blood pressure (thank you, mom), unstable blood-sugar levels and borderline high bad cholesterol levels (again, thank you, mom). We agreed on a plan of action calling for Tracy to have more lab tests, and the doctors looked intently at the results.

A new item that showed up as a result of the lab tests was something called "Chronic Kidney Disease." Tracy had never, as far as I knew, had any difficulty with his kidneys. The doctors explained that the blood vessels servicing the kidneys were similar to those servicing the brain. Chronic high blood pressure does a number on blood vessels, changing them from supple, elastic open tubes, to hard and brittle straws. While Tracy may feel no symptoms, this is another dark cloud hanging over his head. Even though everyone was attempting to lessen dosages where they could, the doctor wanted Tracy to maintain a consistent lower blood pressure, and the only way that could happen was with pharmaceutical help.

I kept reminding them of his medical record: he had an enlarged heart as a result of chronic high blood-pressure; when the doctors at OHSU radically dropped his blood pressure, his heart went into atrial fibrillation, so Tracy's personal optimum blood pressure was almost certainly higher than the norm. One blood pressure medication was working well even when the others were reduced, but the doctors wanted still more of a stable drop. Each time they tried another medication, Tracy didn't do well. He struggled with dry mouth, greater difficulty talking, even more wobbly balance, headaches, mental fuzziness and his regular bugaboo, nausea. During this period of trying new medications, Tracy and I added a question for him each morning after we took his blood pressure: "On a scale of 1-10, how are you this morning?" When I consider what Tracy had to go through just to understand the idea of a "scale" and to conclude where he was on it, it's no wonder that he literally sweated out the answer at first. I had told him it was important to provide a measurement for the doctors so he could reduce the medication he was taking. That he understood and supported. Near the last of November 2011, I noted in Tracy's daily journal, "…T. rates himself as being a 4 out of 10 today. He began taking two Clonidine tablets last night. Very dry mouth, difficulty talking, wobbly balance. He said he had a slight headache yesterday, but said he'd rate himself as being a 6 out of 10 yesterday."

Tracy was prepared to be a guinea pig if it got him where he hoped to be. The odd thing was, in most instances, the medication exacerbated his BP; it didn't make it go down. This trial-and-error scenario went on for many months. Finally, we were able to reduce the number of pills he was taking each day, and some of the dosages, as well. And, while going no lower, his cholesterol didn't go up, either. We also were able to reduce the diabetic blood tests to one a day and then over time stop them altogether. He continues to be tested every few months for diabetes and chronic kidney disease. Visits to the doctor and the lab were pretty common in the first several months Tracy was living at our house. That alone was a big change from his former life. As far as I knew, he rarely saw a doctor and he never had medical tests. Our family culture didn't align itself with going to the doctor unless we were sick, really sick. If nothing seemed wrong, it was not on our radar. We didn't sit around and wonder if something we couldn't feel or see might be wrong. Until something hurt, we ignored it. The concept of "check-ups" was totally foreign. Doctors were for situations like my sister's brain cancer, not visiting them for no apparent reason.

I wanted a regular schedule for Tracy because there were so many things that had to fit into the daily fabric of our lives. Not having a schedule was chaos. Bill didn't see why he couldn't do the things he wanted to do first on any given day and then emerge from his home office and announce it was time for Tracy to walk. Bill is a world-class futzer. He fiddles and futzes and whiles away time doing all sorts of things very important to him and not so important to anyone else. Instead of walking up-and-down the hallway a few times around 10 a.m., often it was closer to noon when he was ready to help out and by that time we were into other exercises or close to being finished or Tracy was resting. Bill would see Tracy sitting in his easy chair and conclude he wasn't doing anything important. In fact, he was resting and didn't need to be disturbed at that moment. Alison and I adjusted. When it worked out for Bill to walk with Tracy, that was great. Often, we walked with him instead. Bill always was surprised when he offered to walk Tracy and found it was already done.

By December, we decided to try walking at a local mall. I thought maybe the act of having to be somewhere at a certain time might help Bill get on with it. The three of us, Bill, Tracy and I arrived at the mall, got the walker from the back of the car, brought along the pink pig just in case, and went towards the mall. Immediately, Tracy almost fell right outside the car door because the cemented area around the handicapped parking area was so uneven. The ramp area caused him to tip backward. I was right there, but I was surprised. I assumed (bad idea) that because it was an area set aside for people with limited physical ability, it was safe. Not for him. Tracy also had tremendous trouble early on with mall flooring. Not the actual flooring, but the different colors and designs. I had never studied mall floors before, but when I did after Tracy's comments, I could see how they could be a challenge. For example, the entryways are either a different material or different paint denoting the entryway. There are stripes on the floors. Sometimes there are diagrams. Sometimes diagonals. These all looked three-dimensional to him, so he never knew if he was to go up-or-down a stairway, a ramp, a hallway. The floor did not look even or flat to him and radiating strips or bars made him throw up. The pink pig came in handy.

Another interesting thing about malls: they are manmade caverns of discordant sound where fake air blows and people rush by. For almost a year, malls overwhelmed Tracy. After this one visit, we decided to leave them alone for awhile, going back months later just to sit and have a mocha and then leave. After this experience, we changed direction. We stayed at home, deciding to walk again with Tracy around our driveway and immediate sidewalk area, still using the walker. He continued to have trouble turning and changing direction without falling down.

Bill sees the world through his own eyes, as does everyone, and finds it impossible to imagine himself as someone else, or see the world through their eyes. And, he doesn't realize that's how he is. He's just very certain what he would do, if he were in what he perceives to be the same shoes. For example, Bill was unable to walk for months after he tore his quad tendon on each knee (in separate occurrences) and after bunion surgery. He spent months in hard physical therapy and exercise to regain mobility. He knew he had knuckled down and worked hard and bludgeoned his way through all barriers to win. When Tracy was relearning to walk, Bill compared what he had gone through to what he thought Tracy was doing. He knew it could be done and concluded that Tracy just needed to more completely apply himself to the effort. When any of us tried to explain, he brushed it off. Alison commented that what Bill had done was great, but what Tracy had gone through was totally different. She said it was as if someone cut the top off Tracy's head, stuck a blender in his brain, gave it a whirl, and said "Now, let's see what you can do." I don't think Bill ever comprehended the difference.

Inside the house, Alison and I had Tracy doing various calisthenics before lunch. Alison and I talked about it and figured if he breathed in more oxygen, perhaps his fatigue level would lessen. We started with deep breathing exercises because he hadn't taken deep breaths in months. As he sat in the chair, we then asked him to stretch various parts of his body. One shoulder had been giving him trouble for some time. When I asked the doctor about it, he indicated that people in wheelchairs often have shoulder pain because they don't have the opportunity to move them and exercise them the way the shoulder is intended to work. Something as simple as tweaking his shoulder while helping him put on a jacket could also have put his shoulder out of sorts. So, slow stretching and movement were good for his shoulders, too. At first he could do a few leg raises while sitting in the wheel chair. His left leg was noticeably weaker. He gradually added more lifts. We stood him at the kitchen sink and locked the wheel chair right behind him. We stood on each side because he would slowly fall to one side or the other. If we weren't there, he'd have fallen all the way over. After awhile, he could stand hanging on to the sink and not fall over. Then we started having him slide from side-to-side as if he were at a ballet barre, still hanging on to the kitchen counter. When he began, he couldn't look out the kitchen window over the sink without getting sick.

Thanksgiving, 2011 five months after Tracy's "event," was a time of true Thanksgiving. This is the one holiday a year where my entire side of the family gets together: my son and his son and daughter, my daughter and her daughter, Tracy and Bill and me. This year was the same, but so different. We all planned to gather once again at our house.

Because we had added Tracy's easy chair to the rest of the furniture in the family room, there wasn't enough room to sit around the fully-extended dining room table for dinner. I decided on a simple and obvious solution: we should move the dining room table into the living room. There was more space and we could more easily accommodate Tracy's wheelchair and the nine other people who would be coming to dinner. Bill resisted. He couldn't see why we had to go to all this trouble rearranging the furniture, as he saw it, just for Tracy. Bill likes me around, in part, because I am independent. But that is a two-edged sword, I also decide what I am going to do with regard to Tracy and the actions I take, based on that decision, often, in Bill's view, disrupt his life and space. Once he complained to my kids "Your mother likes Tracy best." My kids looked at each other and started to laugh. One asked the other, "When did he figure that out? We've always known it. Tracy might as well be her first-born child." In fairness to Tracy, he never vied for the role. Once again, Bill's solution was not to adapt but to rigorously hold tight to his previous "real" life that seemed to have been waylaid and would be back as soon as he could force it to be so – and it was, right after dinner.

At some point on Thanksgiving morning, everyone at the house, except Bill, decided it was the right time to move the table into the living room. This table is Alison's teakwood dining table. It's lovely and I always fear damaging it. The simple and obvious solution quickly became impossible, which Bill more than a little gleefully pointed out. We tried every way possible to move the table past the refrigerator and through the doorway into the living room. Bill held up his end, trying to move and wiggle the table through the opening. There was no way this was going to work. I called my son, Mitch, and asked him to bring his socket wrench. We needed it to make Thanksgiving dinner possible. He laughed.

Tracy held the title of Maestro of Turkey Gravy. This year, I told him someone else would stir it for him, but he was responsible for telling us how much of what to put in when and to check the seasoning. There was quite a committee around the stove top for gravy-making. Both his grand-nieces were in the mix. I'm not sure when a group of people had more fun making gravy. It smelled great and tasted even better. We raised our glasses at dinner to salute many things and one was that Tracy had gotten the gravy right.

Alison's daughter, Nicole, came to dinner and, for the first time since Tracy had his stroke, she saw him face-to-face. The naked happiness on her face read volumes. Also joining us were Nicole's significant other and his daughter. Nicole and Tracy spent time together and she was so obviously relieved that he wasn't as bad as she feared. In the course of the day, we did eat and Tracy tossed his cookies later in the meal, but no one minded. We were eating our Thanksgiving dinner in the living room all together and the day was lovely because Tracy was there.

In early December, my son and I made a flying trip back to Lincoln City to bring "home" Tracy's vehicle, Luna. It had been in Robin's garage since summer along with many of Tracy's other household goods. We asked her if she was planning to use the vacated space for her car and she laughed. No, she was going to use it to store craft supplies. So we brought Luna back to stay first at our house and, later, at Mitch's house. After talking with Tracy, I added my name to the car title. It made sense because we wanted to insure it under our policy. Besides, he was unable to drive it. It was preferable for Luna to move to Mitch's place because she would rest behind a locked gate, and Mitch is a neat freak when it comes to cars and trucks: he takes superb care of them. I asked him to care for Luna, and to drive her on occasion just to remind her what she had been born to do.

About the same time, we picked up several of Tracy's paintings from a Portland gallery that had them in storage but not on display. Bill loaded them in the back of the car and took them back to Lincoln City to the storage unit. While he wasn't as interested in helping with therapy and meals and walking, he was willing to step in to take care of things that could be planned ahead of time, like moving paintings and driving to Lincoln City.

As with many families, the Christmas Holidays are special to us. Everyone has had bad times at Christmas, including us, and Bill and I always work to have a "No Drama Christmas" at our house. We agreed early on that whatever one of us wanted to do was fine with the other one. No justification for any action, however bizarre, was required. Because we give ourselves permission to do anything we want to do, we actually behave rather tamely. Both our childhood Christmases were laden with parental shortcomings: guilt about not enough money for presents, too many unreal expectations, and excessive alcohol which fueled fights. Today, we go for "stressless" holidays and the way we do that, partly, is Bill, the social director, fills the time with many happy things to do. We see family; our friend, Bob, comes on his regular Christmas visit from Illinois; we attend plays and concerts and go out to dinner. Friends come by. Christmas, 2011 was even busier because already busy regular times were now overlaid with holiday events.

Our days became crazy. For example, Tracy had two hours of different types of therapy in the morning on one side of Portland, followed by a matinee and dinner in another part of town, followed the next morning by more speech therapy. He fell asleep in the car as I drove him from one place to another. On Christmas Day, we enjoyed a great dinner together at home followed by going down the street to our neighbor's house to sing Christmas

Carols. Tracy didn't sing, but he grinned. We saw our kids and grandkids around their busy schedules. Mitch is a wonderful dad. I worried early on because I thought he let his kids run circles around him. But when I asked him why he put up with so much from them, he grinned and said, "I just love them." Well, I certainly understood that!

It was fun to see that across the years, my kids still had special places in their hearts for Tracy. They had a long and colorful history together. He is closer in age to my children than he is to me. He played "Marco Polo" in the pool with them in summertime and "Run-Back" football with them anytime it wasn't raining buckets outside. They, and their children, love swimming and fishing and camping along streams and rivers in our great Northwest forests and meadows. Much of that is due to Tracy, who shared his love of the outdoors with them. I've had the pleasure of seeing my daughter, Alison, in her capacity as a wetland scientist walk into a lush wet meadow or overgrown damp forest and unerringly point out where water was. In his turn, Mitch shared his love for baseball, imbibed from Tracy, with his son who has played baseball now for more than half his life.

I think Tracy slept almost the entire week between Christmas and New Year's. I managed to find time to play some bridge. We topped off the holiday season watching the University of Oregon Ducks in the Rose Bowl on January 2. We had friends over for chili and raucously supported the Ducks.

When our granddaughter, Haylee, was 14 years-old, Bill and I took her with us to Hawaii in January. After his birthday in April, 2010, Haylee's brother, Trenton, began reminding us that he would be 14 in 2011… hint, hint. It seemed only fair, so at the end of January and into February, Trenton and his dad, Mitch, came to Hawaii with Bill and me. We had an absolute ball. They surfed and snorkled and ate and toured and went in-and-out of the ocean innumerable times. I think Mitch's favorite part was leaning back in a lounge chair under an umbrella on Waikiki Beach with bar service close at hand while he watched Trenton frolic in the waves. They saw and felt the magic that is Hawaii in winter. After a tour of the campus, Trenton decided he should attend the University of Hawaii. His dad rolled his eyes.

While we were enjoying the heck out of Hawaii, Alison stayed with Tracy at our house. They had a good time as well. Alison became adept at backing the Prius into the garage next to my car – something I still haven't mastered. They kept up the regular schedule and several friends of the Coast Contingent came to visit to assure themselves that everything was O.K. while we were gone.

Through winter and into the spring of 2012, we found our rhythm. Sometimes it felt as if each day ran into another. We were doing the same things day in and day out, week in and week out. But when we compared the end of a period of time with what things looked like at the beginning, there had been substantial progress. For example, Tracy methodically gained physical strength. He exercised every day. It exhausted him and as he got better at it, he exercised more, and it still exhausted him. But he kept doing it. He read out loud an entire column in the University of Oregon Alumni magazine, put his head down on the kitchen table, closed his eyes and did not throw up. He identified more animals with names that began with "L."

With continuing close oversight by his doctors at Physicians Clinic, we were slowly and steadily reducing many of Tracy's medications. As I noted in an email to a friend that January, "…They have caused him so much discomfort: nausea, dizziness/fogginess, diarrhea, lethargy and more. We can't tell what behaviors are stroke-caused vs. which are caused by medication side effects … He has noticeably perked up; talks more, his sense of humor is back; he's doing therapy with Alison and Bill five days a week and not minding it nearly so much. He's walked up-and-down our hallway by himself with NO help… He's thrown up just twice since December 28th and says he'd rather do that on occasion than take the meds that make him feel awful … Another welcome improvement: his senses are regenerating, most of them appropriately. Light and sound don't bother him nearly as much. Smell, however, is interesting. One day he likes something, the next, it smells awful to him…" As to obtaining medical explanations about the side effects to the medication that so bothered Tracy, the doctors listened to all our descriptions of how he acted and felt, nodded sagely and offered two opinions: "That's really interesting," and, "Strokes cause all sorts of problems and we don't know if the side effects are from the strokes he's had or if he would have had problems with side effects in any case.' My conclusion: they don't know.

We slid into regular Wednesday noon meetings at the free Legacy Speech Clinic, beginning in January 2012. For whatever reason, Daria said we were approved to come to another speech therapy visit the next day – a process we repeated for the next three Wednesdays in January before the spigot was again turned off for speech therapy. We never knew why the additional sessions were approved, but we considered each of them a gift.

Tracy isn't much of a groupie. He doesn't often go to meetings or join strangers coming together for some generic reason. I think going to sit with a bunch of strangers bringing with them their various difficulties in a room for an hour at a "speech clinic" was not something he longed to do … at first. With very few exceptions, we went to Daria's speech clinic every Wednesday for nineteen months. Sometimes, Alison and Bill came with us. People who gathered there often came with caregivers, although some were alone. Some made tremendous sacrifices to get there by traveling hours on a bus or waiting hours to get a medical taxi. Some were young with head traumas; some were older with strokes. The common denominator was speech. The shared warmth and caring came from Daria. She brought her own wealth of information and genuine care for anyone who showed up at the clinic. She also brought in students, who learned from people needing help. We all learned the complexities of the many permutations of speech and swallowing. Speech is much more complicated than I ever considered. Just the parts of the brain, where it resides or is controlled, are an amazingly intricate system. There isn't just a one-stop shop for all things speech-related. I recalled the medical information I'd been given by Tracy's doctors and the folks at Forest Grove Rehabilitation Center and the Rehabilitation Institute of Oregon (RIO). In the speech clinic, I saw "real" people with "real" lives struggle with a crazy assortment of speech and cognitive difficulties -- either their own or belonging to the person they cared for.

Tracy continued to struggle with aphasia, a disorder that results from damage to parts of the brain dealing with language. According to information I read, an estimated twenty-five to forty percent of stroke survivors get aphasia. Tracy struggled with speaking, reading, writing, and word retrieval. His difficulty with naming an idea or putting words to an idea continued. He was unable to comply when asked to name a bunch of different fruits, but he could name the one placed before him. He had trouble following fast speech. I've been known as a speed-talker all my life, so slowing my speech was a major adjustment. At a very basic level, he knew what he wanted to say, but he couldn't find the words. At this point, we were definitely not talking about anything as high level as describing a story plot or chaining sequences of events together. Those activities were way beyond his ability. Trying to express his thoughts through writing also was definitely beyond him at this point. Not only could he not find the words he wanted, trying to focus on a piece of paper nauseated him, and his right hand curled and jerked when he tried to control it to write.

When he first attended the speech clinic, he resisted doing anything on the computer even though there were several programs available to assist him with words, and speed and accuracy of thought and action. The sound and the highly animated visuals overwhelmed him. Yet again, this was such a change. For years, I called Tracy whenever I had a computer problem. I'd begin the conversation, "Is the computer doctor in?" And he would know I was calling because my computer had gotten the best of me, once again. He was the person who helped me buy my computers and set them up so they worked for me. One of the many ways he had reinvented himself was to become a good web master. He hosted, designed and managed several websites. His own website for his paintings and photographs was beautiful to look at and easy to maneuver. At first, the group agreed to turn down the lights and noise because it so bothered Tracy. Going fast totally frustrated him. What turned the situation around and got him back to the computer was his ability to help others understand how to use the computer. As he sat in that room, often with his head bent and his eyes closed, he heard individuals struggle with using the computer. He extended himself by concluding he could help them with something he realized he knew about and could share. He helped them use the different games and programs and, in turn, the sounds and lights became less bothersome to his senses.

Generally speaking, the outlook for people with aphasia seems random. Some get better; some don't. But in order to get better, they need help. General medical opinion is that language therapy should begin as soon as possible after brain traumas, including stroke, and be tailored to individual patient needs. Rehabilitation with a speech pathologist involves extensive exercises. So, the majority of the people in the speech clinic fell into the category of being unable to get insurance to pay for therapy or treatment, so they received neither extensive nor tailored treatment.

At this point, I must make a comment. On January 8, 2011, U.S. Representative Gabby Giffords was shot in the head in an awful incident in Arizona. I followed her situation more closely than I would have otherwise after Tracy had his stroke the following June. As a member of the U.S. Congress, Ms. Giffords is the recipient of exceptional health care, the kind of health care everyone in this country should have but most do not. I have watched her phenomenal progress through extensive and intensive therapy with a stalwart caregiver, her husband, retired astronaut Mark Kelly, by her side. As I have watched her struggle with issues evidently similar to those faced by my brother, I have cheered for her to speak better and walk more normally. With the superb care she received, she appears to be doing well. I just wish my brother and so many others like him had the benefit of the marvelous medical treatment available in this country, as Ms. Giffords did.

Unfortunately, that treatment was just not available to Tracy. The excuse in his case was that representatives of the Oregon Health Plan decided people with chronic conditions like strokes won't "benefit" from continued treatment such as physical and speech therapy. I believe lack of funding, rather than medical knowledge, drives decisions such as that. Some may say Tracy "should" have had insurance and "should" have chosen a career that would have allowed him to purchase health insurance. Hindsight is 20-20. If we all knew what was in store for us, lots of things would be different. Most of us don't have a "calling." I know I don't. For those who do, respectfully I ask, shouldn't they try to follow the star that leads them onward? I recognize that everything has its price. I believe Tracy has paid his share and then some. About this same time, we watched Alison struggle to get medical treatment for an on-the-job injury. She was covered by Workers' Compensation but was refused the care she needed. Does having insurance coverage actually help?

If aphasia weren't enough, Tracy also struggled with dysarthria. Dysarthria is a motor-speech disorder in which the muscles of the mouth, face, and respiratory system become weak, move slowly, or not at all after a stroke or other brain injury. Tracy suffered from ataxic dysarthria, which is caused by damage to the cerebellar-control circuit, that is, damage to the cerebellum or to the neural pathways that connect the cerebellum to other sections of the central nervous system. Tracy showed signs of this, including articulation (slurred and slow speech, which early on sounded as if he were drunk as a skunk); prosody (where equal and excessive stress is placed on all syllables spoken); and phonation (harsh, explosive speech that sounded strangled or like he needed to clear his throat). He also struggled to swallow without choking. Working through these sorts of difficulties took incredible strength. Tracy was exhausted after speech clinic. I again reminded myself that mental activity is just as stressful and enervating as physical activity for someone who has had a stroke.

While recognizing all of Tracy's difficulties, I noted that many who came to the speech clinic had much higher hills to climb. Some came determined to get better. Others were much more passive and seemed to have given up. They were the ones who came sporadically, often at the urging of family or a caregiver or the facility where they were housed. The ones who seriously wanted to get better kept coming. The unnerving part of it was that some really wanted to get better but were so damaged they couldn't improve. Other circumstances also complicated things, like moving to different housing or losing transportation or a caregiver being absent. I marveled at what caregivers were all expected to handle. Without help, a person who has had a stroke or other brain trauma likely will never make it through the maze of rules and paperwork. Even grocery shopping -- let alone cleaning the gutters -- can be beyond them. Some caregivers leave something to be desired just like some of the folks they care for. One younger woman who had a stroke at an early age had a husband who still wanted her to cook dinner for him every night. One the other hand, one person who suffered from many problems due to his stroke, didn't want his wife to leave his side, ever, not even for a hair-styling appointment which was her one opportunity to sit down, close her eyes and relax for an hour.

One strength of the group in evidence at the speech clinic was their care for each other. While there was great respect for the professionals, everyone sat up straighter and took more notice when one of their own spoke – or attempted to speak. They were willing to try another game or computer program, if one of their own said they liked it or it worked for them. The patience and care around the table were palpable. I purposely never told a survivor what to do about anything when I was there. I was neither a survivor nor a professional. However, as I kept coming to the speech clinic month-after-month, more caregivers would take me aside and ask me if I had dealt with some problem they faced. In several cases, this was the single place they saw people other than trips to various medical facilities. They couldn't leave alone the person they cared for. Respite care is available, but sometimes impractical for people to access. Besides, we had come to know each other and we trusted one another. In some ways, Wednesdays were a social gathering. We knew many of the "regulars" well enough to worry about them when they didn't show up.

When Tracy and I first started going to the speech clinic, he was in his wheel chair. Sometimes, we came through the courtyard in winter. We could have used another door, but in either case, we'd end up in the same place: the hospital dining room. We would back the wheel chair in the door at the edge of the hospital dining room. The combination of hot dogs, mustard, catsup, pickles, and whatever else mixed with an underlayment of cleaning solution gave off a unique odor that Tracy despised. He would hold his breath until we reached the other side of the dining room and went into the hallway outside the room where the speech clinic was held. He never changed his mind. It always smelled bad to him.

He didn't speak much at first in the speech clinic. Daria kept after him in her friendly, happy way, and he thawed. He also was quite taken by one of the graduate students and thoroughly enjoyed her attention. During the nineteen months Tracy went to speech clinic, he graduated from wheelchair to walker to trekking pole to walking on his own two feet. He became quite expert at playing computer-learning games.

Toward the time he would leave the clinic, Tracy was asked to speak (!) at the monthly Stroke Survivors' Group that met at Legacy Meridian Hospital. He worked on what he would say for six weeks. He also completed several twelve-inch by twelve-inch acrylic paintings to share with the group because his topic was Art and Stroke. The room was packed with an eclectic audience of stroke survivors, their caregivers and various professional staff. A few of the survivors were engineers; one was a farmer. Tracy had worked out a good DVD presentation with a staff member so she took care of the mechanical end of showing his work while he talked. Tracy spoke for an hour on art and its influence on him. He was totally exhausted and elated. So were we. A few months later, there was a party on our last visit to the speech clinic. Tracy was genuinely torn. He was excited and sad at the same time.

On another front, I badgered folks at the Seniors and People with Disabilities office for more help for Tracy. At last, one manager I spoke with understood how Tracy had earned his living. He asked if Tracy's business was still viable. I said I thought it was, that even though he hadn't been able to paint again at the level of his previous work, earlier paintings still were being rented and a couple had sold. He was enthusiastic about that because it meant Tracy could qualify for a special state program called Employment for People with Disabilities. As a result, he could get better health care to support his continued efforts at self-employment. It also meant that he could receive a small amount of earned income without being tossed off the Oregon Health Plan or Social Security Disability. I understood the income part and appreciated it. But, it also meant he would pay a monthly "participation fee" of one-hundred dollars out of the nine-hundred and fifty-three dollars a month he received in disability payments. I never understood what, exactly, Tracy received in the category of *better* health care. It never changed. He couldn't have an appointment with an eye doctor or go to the dentist. He still couldn't receive regular physical or speech therapy. We kept going for the four evaluations allowed each year. They were the only means to see a therapist that I ever found.

There were some exceptions to our routine. The day after we returned from Hawaii, I took Tracy for a follow-up appointment at the Oregon Health Sciences University (OHSU) Stroke Clinic in the Hatfield Research Center up on "Pill Hill" to see how they thought he was progressing. We again requested a review of his various medications and let them know we were working with his regular doctors at Physicians Clinic. The doctor was pretty impressed with Tracy's progress, said he liked the direction his doctors at Physicians Clinic were taking, and asked what therapy he was receiving. I explained the limitations of the Oregon Health Plan/CareOregon insurance. The doctor said Tracy needed intense speech and vestibular therapy. I again explained the limitations. He wrote a prescription for a vestibular evaluation with one of OHSU's therapists and said to continue going to the free speech clinic. Until then, I had not heard a doctor talk about "neural plasticity." I wouldn't be at all surprised that some medical specialist had brought up that word before, but this was the first time it captured my attention. The doctor said that Tracy was younger than most stroke victims and had been in pretty good shape prior to his "incident." Therefore, it was critical to keep pushing for as much therapy as we could get for Tracy that focused on specific tasks and helped him reroute and rejuvenate the pathways in his brain. It would really make a difference all his life. Potentially, he had the capacity to repair, regenerate and recoup much of what he had lost. Tracy's friend, Allan, who has a Ph.D in psychology, is now in private practice and had been the deputy administrator of a state hospital in another state, wrote me about this time " … The good news is that the human brain appears to continue creating new neural pathways throughout most of the lifespan. Thus Tracy retraining his brain is more than possible … indeed it is likely if he remains persistent and interested (the latter is a key component of creating new neurons) … "

I suddenly realized that Alison and I had inadvertently stumbled into doing the absolute best thing we could do for Tracy: give him problems to solve and encourage him to solve them any way he could -- the old way, a new way or a different way. We didn't care. We had said all along that some of the roads inside Tracy's head either had been blown away entirely or tumbled together in a big mess. We had to assist him to find another way or to build a new way to get from A to B. I told the doctor I found it interesting that when I explained to Tracy why we were asking him to do something specific, Tracy listened intently and tried harder. It wasn't just a set of silly exercises. We told Tracy that doing X translated to being able to do Y. He wanted to do Y so he needed to do X first. A great example was Tracy wanted to stand up straight for long periods and not fall over because he wanted to stand at his easel and paint. It started with leg lifts and standing in the corner with his eyes closed. As non-professionals, Alison and I had our own challenges: we had to figure out what we wanted Tracy to do and then what would help him do it. I was terrified that I might ask him to do something that would hurt him. But I was so lucky: all of Tracy's doctors listened to me and answered my questions. I was able to email them with more questions and they always returned my emails.

Tracy was reinvigorated each time he left an appointment in which his doctors and therapists had praised his efforts and said he had every potential to improve. We left with specific projects to do, and he was willing to do them. At first, he was willing to begin them not today but "tomorrow" because while he got a new lease on life each time he saw medical professionals, he also came away from those appointments totally exhausted. I was almost always able to time appointments to accommodate lunch and a nap afterwards. After his nap, he usually was quiet and once I asked him what he was thinking about. He was reliving what he had heard earlier in the day and examining what it meant for him. He was very deliberative, considering everything he had heard from the medical professionals who were treating him.

On Valentine's Day 2012, I found an answer to a question I never considered before: how many Emergency Medical Technicians (EMTs) could we fit into our bathroom? Tracy had gone into the bathroom, using his walker, after awaking that morning. The door was shut. Bill was in his bathroom. I was in the kitchen on the other side of the house. There was a big crash. Bill got there first, pushed the door open, and picked Tracy up off the floor. Tracy crumpled up again, totally passed out, and both of them sank to the floor. Bill yelled at me to call 911. I did, and at the same time, I ran next door to get our neighbor, Tyler, who is a paramedic. He grabbed his little two-year-old daughter and came right over to our house. He took over with

Tracy while I answered questions posed by the 911 operator. I unlocked the front door. Bill got his clothes on just in time for the five EMTs to walk in the door and down the hall with all their equipment. I made copies of Tracy's medications for them and they were asking a series of questions after placing Tracy on a gurney and hooking him up to all sorts of wires. Tyler's little girl, we call her The Mighty Quinn, stood shyly in a bedroom doorway watching all the activity. I thanked her for loaning us her daddy and she looked up at me with big round eyes and said, "Sure!" The EMTs decided to transport Tracy to Good Samaritan because they were not happy with his response or his heart rate.

They left and we followed them to the Emergency Room. After many tests and a CT scan, they concluded it was not another stroke, which of course was what had panicked me. His blood tests showed low blood-sugar and low blood-pressure, which resulted in making him dizzy and faint. His doctors changed his medications again. They were trying for less medication, which was good. We got him back home later in the afternoon with a bump on his nose, where he hit the bathroom counter, a bruise on his right buttock, and two very banged up toenails. I never figured how he wrenched his toenails, but later we took him to a podiatrist to get them back in shape. He spent the remainder of the day resting. I continued to be amazed at the time and energy we were spending interacting with the medical community. It never occurred to me that we would still be so closely tied to them. Don't get me wrong, I'm immensely grateful for their presence, and quite naïve about thinking Tracy was on a straight-up trajectory toward recovering his health. Setbacks seemed more common than I expected.

During this time, Alison was scheduled for shoulder surgery, finally. Post-surgery, the plan was for Alison to recuperate with us, so we were trying to move her easy chair to our living room because she wouldn't be able to sleep lying down for awhile. We also wanted to pick up her prescriptions so we had them after her surgery. Bill threatened to put out a sign on the front lawn that read "Kroger Recovery Home."

The night before her 6 a.m. surgery, her employer cancelled the procedure, saying they had another two days to appeal her worker's-compensation claim. Her attorney told her to sit tight, not talk to any representative from the company and to plan on having her surgery the next morning. I'm glad she didn't hold her breath. She didn't have her shoulder surgery for another six months. In the meantime, she remained in great chronic pain.

Almost three weeks after we put the wheels in motion for Tracy to see a vestibular therapist (a physical therapist with additional knowledge in the field of "balance"), we went back to OHSU and met Andrea in the High Intensity Physical Therapy area. She introduced herself as "Andy." Again Tracy went through the "let's see what you can do" routine. Walking without assistance, he was unable to follow straight lines painted on the floor and proceeded to wobble around the various exercise machines, giving the wall a glancing blow and falling onto tumbling mats before Andy calmly said, "O.K., let's sit here."

We saw Andy for two more sessions in 2012 before we were denied further visits by CareOregon and the Oregon Health Plan. We then saw Andy three times in 2013 before Tracy again was denied further treatment by CareOregon and the Oregon Health Plan. The reason was consistent: they deemed his condition chronic since he'd had his stroke more than six months previously, and they concluded that he would not benefit from further therapy. When medical professionals sought approval from CareOregon to treat him because they saw great potential for improvement, their applications were denied. In two years, Tracy had access to a vestibular specialist a mere six times, even though balance problems and dizziness were paramount on a long list of medical issues he faced. We warned Andy we would have very limited access to her and that Tracy would likely be cut-off with little notice, so we had to make the very most of every minute. We did. Andy not only watched Tracy like a hawk and drew competent conclusions about his current situation, she provided detailed home exercises and was totally reachable via email. Over two years, she and I corresponded regularly in updates and, later, Tracy sent her short emails as well.

About this time, I had written to Tracy's friend, Allan, railing against the insurance limitations for therapy for Tracy. He responded,

"… I'm glad to hear that Tracy is still persevering. I'm sure it must be daunting at times, considering all the factors, not the least of which (and most insidious in my estimation) are the insurance limitations! As a species, we've done a marvelous job of ensuring failure in so many facets of our society and daily lives. We decide the limits of our abilities, even in the face of evidence to the contrary. I find myself disgusted more often than not, and do wonder how we managed to be the animals that flourished to dominate the planet? And yet, here we are. With all the great minds and creativity this world holds, I have to think if anyone of meager intellect were asked how she/he would design the world if the opportunity arose to have a second crack at it, surely that individual would design something better than what we have created! S***, 26 chimps on LSD sitting in front of keyboards could do better by random chance…or maybe that's how we got here…"

Andy took down the walls of the "silos." Up to this point, we were working on specific exercises for specific problems: cognition thinking and memory, eye focus, speech, reading and writing, balance, and strength. She said it was time to come out of those separate "silos" and mix-up various activities. Her first set of exercises for Tracy was interesting … at least I thought they were. Tracy reacted to them with a deep breath, a sigh, and a quizzical look.

Andy liked the walk down the hall, turn and come back exercise. She wanted to add in putting a chair at each end to make a figure eight pattern. She wanted someone at each end of the hallway in the beginning for safety when Tracy turned. We had gone to REI, a great sporting-goods retailer, and Tracy picked out a spiffy-looking trekking pole. He flatly refused to use a cane, so the trekking pole was the winner. He had taken trekking poles with him to Switzerland in his earlier life (how he got them onto the plane with their pointy ends is another story), so he was comfortable using one. We modified the exercise a bit because there wasn't room at one end of the hall for a chair. Instead, we had him turning and wandering into and out of various bedrooms and then back into the family room. When the weather was nice, the exercise became a road show: back to the driveway with the Gelato cones.

Andy offered specific suggestions for increasing stride length and speed as Tracy became more confident and his ability to control his balance grew. Then it got extremely interesting: she added what she called "divided-attention tasks." No more just walking. She said that at the same time he was walking, she wanted him to make a list – out loud – of items at the grocery store, book titles, beverages, or he could recite the alphabet or speak progressions of numbers, skipping every other one.

She added other dual motor tasks – such as taking keys out of his pocket while walking – at the same time still working on his lists. Andy gave him a second circuit as well. It was a step up from standing at and walking along the length of the kitchen counter. She had him take lunges forward, backward, and from side-to-side. Then she added the dual tasks: name occupations, ingredients in a recipe, all the plants he could see outside the window. These skills were clearly designed to rebuild mind and motor skills.

At first, she asked for just ten minutes of practice on each circuit every day or every other day. That was all Tracy could manage at the beginning. The sweat poured out of him as he struggled to concentrate on the given tasks and control his body. He shook with exertion. He fell into doors and the refrigerator. He couldn't complete a list of anything.

Each time Andy and I corresponded via email, I had Tracy read the messages. At the beginning, he couldn't finish one before he was nauseated. But he kept exercising and reading. Within a month, he had added, on his own, two-pound weights strapped onto his ankles as he walked up-and-down the hallway and he increased the number of repetitions to four and then six. One day, I asked Tracy to name all the colors he could think of on the final lap of his walk. He named eight, but they weren't the regular colors like blue and red. They were colors like ochre, cadmium orange, and puce. He began to tell us how and where the colors are made. He got so he held the trekking pole while he walked but didn't use it until he reached the corners. He hated turning corners. He became quite adept at using either the trekking pole or just touching a wall with his fingers to keep his balance as he turned. This was progress! He used to have no idea where he was in space and now he knew.

Outside was a whole different ball game. He had to adjust to bigger space, light, distractions and noise. Outside, I think because the whole perspective is different, he fell more often, but he became increasingly adept over time at a tripod-stance: when Tracy realized he was falling, he would spread his legs and, as he fell, place one hand on the ground to keep from falling completely down. He even perfected the "mini-tripod" stance: in the hand he used to balance, he also held his phone and placed two fingers on the ground, so his hand was a mini-tripod, mirroring his body. Before he got to that point, though, Alison took him walking behind his wheel chair on longer neighborhood walks. Before they went for a walk, they would decide what sort of walk they were taking: balance and finer-motor skills were tested using the walker or the trekking pole; endurance called for walking areas of the neighborhood behind the wheelchair.

On one fine spring day, they decided to take a longer walk without the wheelchair. Tracy had noted the difference between striding and leaning forward on a wheelchair when he walked. He very much preferred striding. I took the opportunity to do some early spring weeding in the front garden. I noted the time they left. I kept checking my watch. They were gone for too long, in my estimation. I looked up-and-down the block and didn't see them. I called Alison's phone. It rang in the house. Great.

As I stood pondering what to do, a stranger came running toward me. The young man ran right up to me and pretty much out of breath, said, "A man has passed out on the sidewalk up the street, and the woman with him asked me to come find you. Do you know them?" My heart skipped more than one beat. I asked him where they were. He took off running with me in pursuit. I found them two blocks away. Alison was sitting on the ground with Tracy's head cradled in her lap. He was awake but definitely not alert. He had tossed his cookies for the first time in awhile. I thanked the young man for finding me and then ran back home to get the car. We loaded Tracy into the front seat and got him back home. That completed his exercise for that day. The combination of a warm spring day and going farther than they planned caused him to crash and burn. He just ran out of steam and collapsed. When Alison saw that Tracy was getting flushed and wobbly, she reached for her phone. She said she couldn't believe that she'd left her phone at the house. That never happened again.

A week later, on another nice day, Alison and Tracy again went walking outside. It was a repeat performance: Tracy passed out, fell, vomited, and was very disoriented and tired for the rest of the day. Alison again cradled him as he went down, so he was not hurt. I worried more about her and her shoulder because I knew she'd put herself in harm's way before she let harm come to Tracy. That time, Bill came to the rescue.

We saw the doctor a few days later and brought up what had occurred, twice. After another CT scan, the doctor said that when Tracy was exhausted, it was an instant condition, not a gradual one. In time, hopefully he would learn to read the signs of exhaustion before he fell in a heap. One step we took was to put a pedometer on Tracy, asking him to monitor the distance he walked. We also asked him to stay in his wheel chair until after breakfast due to his usual greater dizziness when he first got up. I was interested in my own aplomb now. I no longer fell into my own mental heap when Tracy fell. I had become more matter-of-fact over things that used to toss me for a complete loop.

By the end of March 2012, Tracy was walking five days a week, outside preferably early morning or late afternoon, out of the heat of the sun. He used the trekking pole more and the walker less. At first, I reminded him to look up and focus on a point farther away when he walked, not look at his feet, and to take longer strides instead of little shuffling steps. He concentrated on looking farther ahead.

Andy told us that building on the dual and, ultimately, triple-task idea (walking, making a list, and taking something in-and-out of his pocket) was crucial to help his brain regenerate. She said he might find it impossible at first to do all we asked, but to persist. The act of walking, according to her, will take up residence in the higher brain centers after a stroke and that function is perfectly happy to reside there permanently unless we work to move it back again to the more automatic centers. The divided attention tasks help to accomplish this. Andy acknowledged that this was hard work, and that the exercises needed to be interesting and challenging. She reiterated that the cognitive tasks were forcing walking to become more automatic and that it's very hard work cognitively to move walking away from conscious thought to the more automatic part of the brain. She praised efforts at consistency of practice because this was the key to making and strengthening new neural connections. At first the connections are somewhat fragile and need repetition to become robust and automatic. Tracy took to the walking with simultaneous mental tasks better than he did to the kitchen sink lunges. Those wiped him out, I think because he expended great energy keeping track of balance and where he was in the space around him.

About this time, I asked Tracy to critique his progress. He said his legs were getting stronger and he was more at ease with the trekking pole. He observed that tight turns were just as hard as ever. He said he appreciated Andy's efforts, but said that while he was working to accommodate his balance/dizziness, it was no better. Left to itself, the balance/dizziness problem caused him to tip or fall over the same way it had since his stroke. However, he said that the accommodations we were all trying (walking, the trekking pole, weights, etc.) helped him to walk and that was good. He and I wistfully dreamed about how nice it would be if, someday, a light bulb went on and he was no longer dizzy or out of balance. He said until that time, he was willing to work hard at finding and using accommodations. He also trusted Andy when she told him that with continued practice she believed it was possible to build a strong system around the dizziness so that over time it would have less impact. Challenging the dizziness to the degree possible through exercise to regenerate or create new neural pathways made it less easily triggered. At this point, it made more sense to aim for a higher threshold rather than to hope the problem magically disappeared.

A month later, Tracy still was wearing two-pound weights and had added a pedometer app on his iPhone. He was interested in extending his mileage. He still was adjusting to the challenges of walking outside: bigger space, more light, distractions and noise. People stopped and wanted to talk because they had seen him every day and noted his progress. At first, he found it hard to stop the movement of walking, stand still, focus on a close-by face, and talk. We would thank our neighbors for their care and move on. Later it became much easier, and Tracy came to love chatting and became a regular dog petter. People who walk their dogs like to have people admire their pets. Tracy is built for that job.

When asked, Tracy said he always was dizzy. It got worse when he turned his head or his body. When he turned corners during his walking exercises, we had him count by two's. Interestingly, he generally remembered where he left off between turns; he didn't have to begin again. We began to ask him to discuss, rather than merely name, colors. He retained detailed knowledge of the colors he uses for painting and he told us how he mixes them. Sometimes we'd ask him to name all the cities in Europe that he visited. He had great recall of things further back in memory. He was getting better at short-and mid-term memory but it was an effort. We saw Andy once more early in June 2012. The next time we saw her was almost a year later. Meanwhile, we stayed in touch via email.

In early spring, Tracy began to watch TV. Instead of sleeping in front of the TV, all of a sudden, he was watching shows on science, engineering, cooking, law and order, travel, history, DIY projects, and racing cars, and he knew the twists and turns in each of them. He was using Netflix like a crash course to get up to speed with the world. We took him to movies, and a play, and out to dinner, and he did fine.

At the last of March 2012, I asked Tracy if he would like to go with me to Lincoln City for a couple of days. It would be his first trip home since he left his house one afternoon in June 2011 to go to the gym. He said he wanted to go but was worried that he couldn't handle a big crowd of people. I promised we'd limit the numbers and the times he saw folks, telling them Tracy would be back again, soon, especially if the first trip was a success. He managed the longer driving trip well, in part because he closed his eyes and rested by sitting very still for portions of the drive.

I practiced what my dad taught me many years ago: drive, swerve, turn, stop and start as if I had eggs loose in the car and didn't want to break them. We stayed at Chef Sharon's house, and I think the most fun Tracy had was with her two cats, Earl Grey and Crumpet. He hadn't seen them since they visited him at the Forest Grove Rehabilitation Center the previous summer. On Saturday, he received a massage with his beloved Faith, and I participated in a hands-on pasta cooking class with my friend, Sharon.

Tracy enjoyed surprising more friends when he went with us to the Bay House where Evans and Jim and other friends in the Hot Club du Jour band were playing music in the lounge on Saturday night. Tracy loved the stir he created when he walked in, leaning on my arm. He wanted to be on his own two feet, not using any mechanical devices, when he saw his friends again on his home turf. The first one to see and recognize him stood up from her chair at a small cocktail table, gasped and pointed. Others around her turned to see what had gotten her attention. In turn, they stood and clapped. Members of the band were just setting up. They left the stage and gathered round. That was a very happy evening. We visited the Beach Dog Café for breakfast on Sunday and again, we surprised a multitude of folks, which he loved. So many told him that the Coast was a little brighter with his presence. He told them all that his main goal was to return home. Tracy slept more for most of the next week to recoup from his great trip after we returned home to Beaverton.

I spent the day after we returned home with Alison in mediation about her shoulder. It took all day and was not pleasant. The result was that she was supposed to get her shoulder repaired. I kept thinking her employer had a big fat attorney, consultants, and deep pockets, and Alison had her mother and an attorney with one foot out the door to retirement. After the economic downturn in 2008, Alison was unable to get enough work in her professional field of environmental consulting, so she was taking whatever jobs she could find. One was at a national grocery-store chain. Alison had injured her shoulder at work lifting and moving large, heavy racks of bread from the loading dock into the store. She did the work as instructed and as she was trained. After her injury, she found other employees had had similar injuries. The company changed the way it stocked bread after Alison's injury. She was moved to another job in the store, that of checker, where she was still required to lift and bag heavy items such as gallons of milk. She did eventually have her surgery in August 2012, but the company refused to pay for the post-surgery physical therapy she needed. After the operation, her shoulder has never been the same. Each time I pass where she worked, I curse the store. I will never, ever buy groceries, or anything else, from them ever again. Tracy was concerned about Alison, as well, and the two talked about how to get along in this world when you are not quite as fit as you want to be.

Later in April, I attended a five-day "French Cooking Intensive" class in Lincoln City, spearheaded by Chef Sharon. I stayed with Tracy's friends, Matt and his Tracy, using Wonderful Harry's bedroom because he was away at college. I remember the big poster of Che Guevara on his ceiling.

Lincoln City has a Culinary Center on the fourth floor in the same building as City Hall and the Library. Cooking classes and demonstrations are offered for a fee to the public. Usually, the classes are a few hours, or a day. The intensive French cooking class was special, exhausting, exhilarating, tasty and a complete change of pace for me. I loved it. Each day had its own menu overseen by Chef Sharon. Class members were expected to prepare, plate and, of course, eat. I and my classmates became familiar with a map of France and learned to cook by region and season. We learned to pair wines with food. Our mouths were full of the words and flavors of "Coquilles St. Jacques, soufflé, mesclun avec vinaigrette, omelette Arlequin, galette," and more. Our hands made baguettes and crème brulee and crème a la glace aux pruneau (plum ice cream). One of my personal joys is going to cooking classes and this one was superb. I met Sharon's friends, Liz and Sally, who taught the class, and I worked my tail off getting involved in everything we cooked. I'm so appreciative of Bill and Alison for making it possible that I could take the class. I've enjoyed much pleasure cooking for family and friends since. Tracy didn't mind, either! Later, in the warmth of summer, two "foodie" friends came over and we made soufflés. Tracy helped.

In early May, Tracy's friend, Matt, came to town and we three trooped to the Portland Art Museum to take in the Rothko Exhibit. Mark Rothko is considered one of the most famous post-World War II American artists, an abstract impressionist, and one of Tracy's favorites. My take when I saw his work was, wow, this stuff is big! Tracy was still using his wheelchair for these sorts of excursions and I found it interesting that he moved as far away from the painting as the room allowed. He said the size and the fact that he moved his head up-and-down and side-to-side to view an entire painting made for a nauseating experience. However, he wanted so much to see the exhibition, he conquered the nausea. That was a first. Up to now, he had done something until he threw up. This time, he worked his way through the nausea.

Sometimes that meant he sat there very quietly with his eyes closed. But then, he'd open them again and move on. When I first saw him facing the front of the exhibit and realized his eyes were closed, I thought, that looks funny: someone looking at something with his eyes closed. Never again will I make assumptions when I see someone looking at something with their eyes closed. Tracy taught me to what lengths one must go to conquer nausea. After seeing the exhibit, we ate a late lunch at nearby SouthPark, a favorite restaurant of Tracy's, and had a delicious time. Each time I saw Tracy in a setting with his friends, he was coming more alive, more animated, more here in the present. It was lovely to experience.

Chapter 3:
The Living Room is an ... Art Studio

In early summer 2012, we expanded the definition of "living" room. We decided to make it into a space Tracy could use for living and exercise, hence several pieces of furniture would have to go. Actually, except for company, I was the only one who sat in that room. In the past, I enjoyed watching the late afternoon light on the garden and spent time there reading and listening to music. There hadn't been much time for any of that in the past year.

Evans, of Hot Club du Jour fame, loved the idea of restoring our grandmother's melodeon (a small reed pump organ housed in rosewood and powered by a system of bellows and pedals) and took it to his music store in Newport. So there it went. The heavy hide-a-bed couch went away, too. After seeing Tracy's success with Wii at speech clinic, we borrowed the interactive equipment from my nephew, Trenton, so Tracy could watch the TV screen and virtually ski, roll, bowl and participate in lots of other sports. Those activities required space, at least in the beginning, because he frequently fell sideways and we made sure he fell into something that didn't hurt him.

We brought Tracy's TV from Lincoln City to Beaverton, putting it into our living room. Tracy was rapidly expanding the repertoire of what he watched on TV. I thought it interesting that he crossed the threshold of watching "how to" TV to viewing live TV: mostly sports. Bill complained that Tracy watched things on TV (particularly sports) that he didn't like, so this was a good chance to put Tracy's TV in the living room, leaving the TV in the family room for Bill. Of course, Bill never left his office/bedroom to watch TV during the day, but he said he might want to and couldn't with Tracy watching our TV in the family room. I figured he was just complaining. It was more important for Tracy to get better at the pace he was on than worry about whether Bill might want to use the TV for something other than sports. I enjoy sports, too, so it was fun to watch baseball during the summer and football in the fall with Tracy. We all managed to find something to watch in the evening together that we enjoyed.

In due course, Madeline and Doug, friends of Tracy's from the coast, came to the rescue, transporting items Tracy identified as necessary to set up his studio. When Madeline heard what we were trying to do with the living room -- and that we planned to rent a truck to bring some of Tracy's things to our house -- she said, "Well, finally, here's something we can do for you." Doug had the cleverest truck that he used to bring all the varied stuff Tracy needed. An enclosed small truck, it had shelving at the sides and straps strategically hung on the inside of the roof, making it efficient for transporting a wide assortment of items. Madeline rode shotgun and was welcome in and of herself, but she also is the creator of the best chocolate-chip cookies I've ever eaten! Paul -- our steadfast friend the contractor -- installed shelves, floors, lights, work benches, and the easel. I noted with quizzical aplomb that Paul laid down pieces of plywood over the living room carpet – and then screwed them down so they wouldn't slip. I bet that rug never thought it would be screwed to the floor! A new lighting system was installed over the easel. Tracy thought his old one was perfectly fine, but Paul deemed it a fire hazard and refused to put it up. Tracy never agreed, but gave in.

The exercise routine continued through spring and into summer. Tracy added more distance to his walks. He walked more with the trekking pole and less with the walker. He could read a column in the University of Oregon alumni magazine and retain what it said without throwing up. His lunges at the kitchen sink were more controlled and he could manage more of them at a time. He talked more. There were pleasant asides too, like the time Sharon, Tracy's chef friend from Lincoln City, stopped by and had us make big, puffy pretzels. Tracy was up to his elbows in dough. He found the twisting and shaping of the pretzels to be a challenge, but his looked better than mine did. We ate them all!

We joined in the celebration of a new "Sunday Trailways" event in which the local Tualatin Hills Park and Recreation District showcased the opening of a link in the nearby Fanno Creek Regional Trail. Several local trail lovers, myself included, had worked for years to achieve this success. Tracy came to the event, and Alison and I pushed him in his wheel chair along the new route on a lovely spring day enjoying gorgeous landscape views and a bald eagle in a tree. Tracy and I were interviewed earlier in the year by the

Beaverton Valley Times, a local weekly newspaper, which ran an in-depth article about both of us headlined "A Change of Plans." We were again interviewed on this "Sunday Trailways" day and were able to share how much Tracy had progressed. Tracy was great in these interviews. We talked together prior to both of them so he knew what to expect. He said if sharing his story could help anyone who had suffered a similar "event," he was happy to do an interview a week!

We celebrated my birthday, June 10, with Tracy and friends at my favorite restaurant, the Joel Palmer House, in Dayton, Oregon. We were there the previous year just ten days before Tracy's stroke. That seemed a lifetime ago, and yet, the same people were at the table. We laughed and had a grand time. During the summer, friends came to visit Tracy from Nevada. Allan and Carol, Tracy's friend of long-standing and his so-talented violinist wife, came to check up on him as did Ed and his wife, Kris. Ed is a friend from high school days.

We took another jaunt to the Portland Art Museum, this time to see a Monet exhibit. Tracy, Alison and I (well, I most of all) had been enthralled by Monet's garden in Giverny, France, a few years prior, and wanted to see paintings that reflected his love of his garden. And, Alison finally had her shoulder surgery in August. She stayed at our house for a week in her easy chair in our living room. Five days after the surgery, Bill's oldest grandson, Kade, age twelve, came to visit from the Chicago area. He stayed a week. He and Bill went on many adventures, so I didn't see much of either of them. Kids are great. Kade took one look at who was living at our house and what shape they were in, and just kept on trucking. Nothing fazed him. We might think we were a bit unusual, but he took it totally in stride.

For the first time since Tracy's "event," I hosted a table of bridge in our "living room." The bridge table and chairs fit quite well on the plywood flooring after we rolled the work benches to the side. My friends said they'd played bridge in many places over the years, but never in an artist's studio, so we added another experience to our lives! The ladies loved visiting with Tracy, and he appreciated being able to put faces to the names I had tossed about in various conversations over the past several months.

After the success of Tracy's initial visit to Lincoln City in March 2012, we began planning for another trip toward the end of June, about a year after his "incident." We again stayed at chef Sharon's home and, this time, Alison joined us. I asked Tracy to specify what he wished to accomplish on the trip.

He said he was ready to take a look at where his things were. He knew they were in Robin's garage, at Sharon's, and in a storage unit, but he was ready to look inside and take some pictures.

We were invited to Rosie's. For a few years, Evans, who led Hot Club du Jour, and his band of talented musicians had practiced on Monday evenings at Rosie's place, a sumptuous bed and breakfast in a great old house overlooking the Pacific Ocean in Lincoln City. She hosted the Monday evening practices, and significant others and friends would bring food (extremely good food!) and wine and play Skipbo (a crazy card game) while they listened to the musicians playing in the other room. Tracy had been part of this social event, and we heard often from members of the group and Rosie about how they – and Rosie's cat -- missed him on Monday nights. So, Tracy said he'd like to go back to Rosie's for an evening of friendship and music. We weren't going to be there on Monday, so the whole group moved their practice and dinner to Thursday night.

Tracy wanted to see Heidi's Sea Creature, as well. Heidi, one of Tracy's artist friends, was in the throes of finalizing the creation of this enormous metal sculpture. It was still in her barn and she was pondering how to get another hoist to put its head on. Her hoist was too short. This is one big Sea Creature! Subsequently, the Sea Creature was placed with great fanfare in its new home overlooking Devil's Lake from Regatta Park in Lincoln City. In a naming contest, local school kids decided to call the Creature "Sparky," a grand name for a sea dragon. Heidi asked the children and other community members to write their greatest wishes on small pieces of paper that she then put into Sparky's heart. Many, many heartfelt wishes for Tracy found their way into Sparky's heart.

Besides fulfilling Tracy's desire to see the Sea Creature, Heidi and her husband, Dave, put together an evening barbecue at their Barking Dog Organic Farm on a soft Saturday night. We had superb lamb and sat around a big fire outside under the grape arbor as it gently rained around us. Many of Tracy's friends were there. I watched some of them gently touching him, just to be sure he was really there. Others were content to sit and look at him. Heidi wrote after the visit, "…Saturday was wonderful…absolutely wonderful. We have all pretty much determined that Tracy is the 'glue' that holds us all together. I hadn't seen many of those wonderful friends in way too long…"

On Friday, the three of us enjoyed an "Italian Small Plates

Demonstration" again under chef Sharon's fine hand at the Culinary Center. On this trip, Tracy was more animated than he'd been in a long time. He made his friends laugh and there was a lot of story-swapping. The trip did Tracy a world of good, and I know his friends loved seeing him, too. This trip was another resounding success, building on the first trip in March.

In late July, Alison, Tracy and I again traveled to Lincoln City for a few days and stayed at Sharon's. This time we "cat-sat" while she was on vacation. Again, we spent an evening at Rosie's, eating great food, talking and laughing, and listening to terrific music. This time it was the regular Monday evening practice night. We talked with Doug, clever truck owner, and Madeline, chocolate-chip cookie expert, about our planned creation of a studio in our living room. They offered to bring the items we needed for Tracy's new living/exercise space when we were ready for them. Subsequently, they delivered a big work table, the materials to reconstruct his easel, various paints, paper and smaller stretched canvasses, tools, his beloved big bed, and his big flatscreen TV. Tracy's couch remained at Sharon's along with his dining-room table and chairs.

During this time, I became an instant expert on something else: glass. Tracy used a piece about 18" x 24" and a little thicker than regular window glass on which he mixed paint. One side he used for acrylic and the other for oil. He would need this in his new temporary studio. Finding an old piece of glass just lying around wasn't that easy. Glass gets brittle over time and recyclers are interested in recycling it, not saving it. For his purposes, Tracy needed real glass, not something like plexiglass. Paul, our friend and contractor came to the rescue. After finding a piece that suited Tracy's needs – not too heavy because he needed to lift and turn it – Tracy taped the edges and pronounced it good.

In September 2012, cousin Roy visited from Philadelphia. It had been too long since we last saw him. Roy and his younger brother, Mark, are the sons of our mother's sister. Their mother spent her life on the East Coast. Tracy's and my mother had moved "Out West" during the Depression, considered by the family, according to her, to have been married to a ne'er-do-well because he hadn't pursued a corporate career. I was age 17 the first time I met my cousins and was returning from an American Field Service exchange-student trip to West Germany. I'm not sure when Tracy first met our cousins, but when we all finally got together without our mothers present, we had a darned fine time. As children, we had gotten the impression that mother hadn't apparently liked her older sister very much. Her sister was named Helen Page, after her mother, Helen, and mom told us that their father dubbed her "Yellin' Rage." Long ago I concluded that my aunt more than likely had a similar level of warmth toward her younger sister. Now, I'm not so sure. Anyhow, it was fun to see Roy and hear about his latest adventures.

Tracy also was visited by Jennifer from the Portland Art Museum's Rental Sales Gallery, where he had several paintings rented or sold over the last few years. Jennifer brought a beautiful bouquet of flowers and her great dog, Lou, for Tracy to pet. Our cats were less than pleased to host a DOG, but he was very polite. Jennifer reiterated that she wanted Tracy to continue to get better, and she looked forward to the time when he would show new art work with her.

Alison once again stayed with Tracy when Bill convinced me to go with him to San Francisco for a few days. We had fun, played tourist, ate good Italian food and didn't speak of things back home.

Tracy completed several doctor's visits through the summer and into the fall of 2012, continuing to try to reduce his medications. At one doctor's appointment, he noted that his neck and shoulders were tight and sore. He was having trouble turning his head – which he tried to do with great care because of his dizziness. I asked the doctor if she thought massages might be a good thing, since Tracy had used them before his stroke to mitigate shoulder and neck issues triggered by standing at his easel for long periods when he painted. She said yes and I began the hunt for a special massage therapist. We needed a nurse because of the intricate difficulties in the back of Tracy's head. In late June, we found Cheryl. She was so very helpful and Tracy so appreciated her ministrations. I took Tracy to see Cheryl every two weeks with few exceptions over the next fourteen months. CareOregon and the Oregon Health Plan did not pay for the massages.

A late August lab report looked promising, showing things pretty much in balance for Tracy. Over the months as he became more aware of himself -- his situation and the world around him -- he sometimes became more "prickly," yelling, slamming the TV remote around if it didn't do what he wanted immediately and beating on his hand when it didn't perform to his expectations. Tracy was frustrated if things didn't go his way on the first go-around. Partly, I think, that was do to his increasing awareness of his status and what his limitations were. Sometimes, he would sink into a quiet funk. Mood swings were evident especially when he was on a "high" from visiting friends, and then he returned to his regular routine.

Way back in the summer of 2011 when he was at Forest Grove Rehabilitation Center, Tracy exhibited signs of depression: gritting his teeth in anger, crying in frustration. The doctor suggested placing him on a low dosage of Zoloft, an anti-depressant. I totally resisted that idea. I wanted Tracy to come back from the fog he was in, not sink deeper into it. I also believed he was strong enough -- with enough help from us -- to make it through the tough times. The doctor was gently insistent. He pointed out that depression is a common and fundamentally debilitating condition that hits stroke victims. He said it could derail any progress Tracy might make. He also pointed out that depression is not some sort of emotional weakness. It's a huge burden to carry for those who have it, and any way that burden can be lessened is good. Subsequently, we agreed to place Tracy on a very low dosage of the common anti-depressant. He remained on it with good effect for more than two years.

I was firm with Tracy that he could not, absolutely not, continue having red rage attacks. Spiking his blood pressure with anger or stress could, in his case, be fatal. We needed to find a way to help him so he didn't get so angry. I told Tracy he was on the anti-depressant and that if he felt a boost in the dosage would help him to avoid bouts of anger, we should talk to the doctor. Tracy followed his natural pattern and digested the information, concentrating on all facets of it. Interestingly, he also talked with Kelly, close friend and fellow artist, about taking the anti-depressant. She urged him to get off it entirely because of her concern, and the concern of many artists, that anti-depressants smother or weaken creative drive and ability. He was caught. He certainly didn't want to weaken his creative juices, but he also got very angry, especially when frustrated.

We asked his doctor about his conundrum. She suggested seeing a "prescribing psychiatrist" or primary mental-health nurse practitioner for evaluation. We pursued this through CareOregon and found Sequoia Mental Health Clinic. In the course of time, he received an evaluation and had a couple of sessions with Ryan. I guess there are some really sick people out there, and I'm sorry. Ryan said meeting Tracy and me was a breath of fresh air. He listened to everything we told him about the frustration and anger vs. Tracy's concern about negating or weakening his artistic creativity. Both he and the psychiatrist who evaluated Tracy said they thought Tracy would do fine without the anti-depressant but that he would need to consider ways to help himself stop being so angry or frustrated. We asked that this information be shared with Tracy's primary-care physician at the Good Samaritan Physicians Clinic.

Then something unexpected happened. He had a new doctor at Physicians Clinic who wanted to review and modify his medications. The doctor suggested reducing the anti-depressant dosage to the lowest level possible, but staying on it because it was acting synergistically with his other medications and provided part of the potassium his kidneys needed.

There were several medical fits-and-starts in the fall. The doctor again tried to change medications and Tracy didn't react well. We wound up going back to an earlier medicine to control blood pressure that had worked well. Tracy still takes a cocktail of four medicines to control blood pressure, so getting them all to behave nicely with each other is a challenge. Finally things seemed in balance at a level the doctor could live with and so that's where it stays. As Tracy has accomplished goals he's setting for himself and he's thought about what he wants to do both as a painter and a photographer, he's been able to sidetrack or derail his anger. As one of his early occupational therapists noted, Tracy is lucky: he has good judgment. He understands the consequences of anger.

Tracy's birthday on October 6 was a quiet one in 2012, as compared to world travels in previous years and the big event of his coming out of "institutional care" and moving in with us the previous year. But it was an appropriate time to reflect on changes experienced over the past year. His alma mater is the University of Washington and, even though he received his masters in fine arts degree at the University of Oregon and he mostly supports the Oregon Ducks, it's hard for him to watch a big rivalry football game like the one presented to him on his birthday: the Washington Huskies vs. the Oregon Ducks. I made no bones who I was rooting for – Oregon, of course! He wished the Huskies well but he knew they were unlikely to win. They didn't. As football seasons came and went, I marveled at how Tracy retained intricate details, history and statistics of the game. That part of his brain had been untouched. We enjoyed birthday cake in spite of football!

Bill took off on his regular jaunt to Reno for several days the day after Tracy's birthday in October. As Alison noted, Bill seemed to have been able to keep his life intact. Nothing much had changed for him. He still kept his same daily and nightly schedule and took the trips he wanted. He kept busy with a social schedule and attending political and current-event forums. Bill might say differently, I believe, but in reality, he wasn't terribly inconvenienced. A common response to me when I asked him to do something was he couldn't see that whatever "it" was, was necessary. He would shrug his shoulders and say, "Well, you're the one who wants to do all these things for Tracy, so if you want to, fine. I don't think you have to provide a Cadillac, but if you want to, that's your business."

Since Bill didn't actually want to know the details of Tracy's situation, he didn't notice regular therapy or clinic appointments. He seemed surprised, for example, when he suggested I join him to do something only to discover that it was at the exact same time as the regular speech clinic.

Bill was amazed at the number of doctor's visits and lab runs involved in Tracy's care. If I pushed him to help, he'd consider it if he could put it in his day planner first. To balance this observation, though, Bill behaved the same way when I asked him to do something about the garden. It wasn't that he didn't like Tracy, or the garden for that matter. It was more that it disrupted his own schedule. Twice, I asked him to take Tracy to the speech clinic. Begrudgingly, he did, but he wouldn't stay in the room. Bill attended meetings four nights a week where he was able to vent as much as he wanted. I figured that helped, but sometimes I wondered what those people must think of me. Later, Bill told me he never once said anything negative about me at his meetings.

Each fall, the Portland Art Museum Rental Sales Gallery puts on a soiree to showcase some of its artists and to highlight coming events for the year. In 2011 four months after his stroke, I went for Tracy. In 2012, Jennifer asked Tracy if he'd like to come, and he said he would. However, he was worried about the crowds and the noise. I suggested we go for a just a little bit; they could introduce him and point out work still available, and then we would go to dinner. Tracy was well received and so many people wanted to talk with him, saying they were very happy to see him. It did his heart good. Afterward we joined friends for dinner at a great little Guatemalan restaurant in Beaverton. Tracy liked that, too.

Instead of just going to an upcoming doctor's appointment, I suggested to Tracy he might want to think of something else he'd like to do nearby. He thought about that and said that Utrecht, a supplier of all things *painting*, was close and maybe we could stop in and buy a few supplies. He enjoyed a good time there, wandering the aisles for the first time in more than a year. He noted price differences from a year or so before, and I thought that was interesting. When we left, we spotted a cute little restaurant. Since we still had time before our appointment, we ate lunch there. It was the first time in a long while that Tracy had been out in Portland not just for a medical reason, and he enjoyed himself.

At Utrecht, he enjoyed leisurely perusing different picture framing materials, brushes and palette knives and paint. He also enjoyed taking his time perusing the lunch menu. We have teased Tracy because when he is looking at a menu to decide what he wants to eat, he closes his eyes and smacks his lips as he contemplates what the specific item might taste like. He took the time to go through that routine in this little mid-Eastern restaurant, which smelled good, and we had a tasty and relaxed lunch.

In the fall of 2012, the doctors and Tracy were less than pleased with progress on the pharmaceutical front. His new doctor wanted his blood pressure, cholesterol and blood sugar to stabilize at lower levels. Each new medication he tried had nasty side effects. Tracy said it was like he was almost feeling good (if he ignored his dizziness) and then he'd get walloped by the old side effects: dizziness, sapping of his strength or his desire to do anything, fuzzy thinking and nausea. Additionally, his blood pressure and blood sugar started going up-and-down like a roller coaster.

We asked if he could return to the old medications he'd been taking because they seemed to work well enough with minimal side effects. I think the doctor wanted to fine tune some more, but Tracy said he'd had enough experimentation for awhile. Tracy didn't want to gain back the weight he'd lost because it was better for his frame and his balance to be lighter. On the other hand, he had developed a real hankering for almost everything sweet. He hadn't really been much of a "sugar-holic" before his stroke, but sweet things just seemed to seek him out afterward.

In November, Tracy and I expanded his horizons a bit further. We went shoe shopping at REI, one of his favorite stores. His shoes were in need of replacement because he'd been walking more outside. With the challenges he had falling and trying to balance himself, his shoes took a beating. They looked as if they had been flattened all along the sides. Arm-in-arm, we went into the store where he stood just inside the doors, closed his eyes and sniffed deeply. He identified the smell of tents, skis, kayaks, hiking gear, and new shoes. Then he smiled, opened his eyes, and we walked directly toward the new shoes on display diagonally across the store. He knew where to go. He'd been in the store before and remembered it.

Tracy handled his transaction. The sales associate worked with him. In all the interactions we had with people "out in the world" after Tracy's stroke, every single person treated him with respect and dignity. They realized that something had happened to him, but they coordinated their pace and their speech to his speed. As he got more comfortable interacting with strangers, he forthrightly told them he had had a stroke. They would indicate dismay, primarily I think because he doesn't fit the generally accepted visual profile of the type of person who had a stroke. Tracy looks pretty youthful and appears to be in great shape. When he searched for a word, he held up his forefinger and said with a smile, "Bear with me, I've had a stroke!" Inevitably, the response was, "Take your time." I believe, based on my experience during this time with Tracy, that people will react well if given a reason to and a chance to. Tracy never acted the victim or requested something unreasonable from a stranger. People responded in kind.

Another Holiday Season was upon us. We had so much to be thankful for. The previous Thanksgiving, Tracy also had been with us, but sitting at the table with the noise and activity flowing around him had been a terrific effort for him. He was exhausted before he got up to the table. But in 2012, before he brought himself to the Thanksgiving table, he helped set it and brought food to it, cracking jokes all the while.

At the table, we had our family, except Nicole, my granddaughter, who was at her boyfriend's parents' home, and we were joined by our great friend, Linda. Linda had moved in to a house down the street three years earlier and we realized over time how lucky we were to have her in the neighborhood.

On Christmas Eve, Bill, Tracy, Alison, our friend Bob from Chicago, and I trooped down to Linda's house once again to sing Christmas carols. Now this is a bigger deal than you might think. Besides being a master gardener, Linda is a retired professional opera singer and college music professor, who plays a mean grand piano. Her dog, Juju (as she explains, the good kind of Juju, not the bad kind) is a warm brown standard poodle who "sings" when she plays the piano. I think he sounds better in the chorus than I do! Over the holiday season, we saw live performances, ate great dinners out, went to movies and still had time to visit and laugh. It set the stage for the "Big Event" we planned in January.

Bill and I had been going to the Hale Koa Hotel in Honolulu for years. Before our first trip, we laughed and said we were getting old: Old People went to Hawaii in the winter. After our first trip, we agreed that we'd had much more fun than we had dreamed possible and promptly made reservations for another trip the next winter. For many years after that, we went to Hawaii almost annually. The Hale Koa is a special place. Its name is Hawaiian for House of the Warrior, and it's open to active duty and retired military. It's not owned by the government, and it's supported by its visitors. Bill made it possible for us all to spend time at the Hale Koa. He said he traded surviving getting shot at while in the Army for a place in the sun. In 2012, he and I had vacationed in Hawaii, taking our son and grandson with us. It was hard to tear myself away because Tracy was still so sick, but Alison stayed with him. Bill convinced me the two of us should get away together. We did, and I had a restful and relaxing time in the sunshine. I always love Hawaii in January. I actually get warm with almost no clothes on! So, in 2013, we decided it was time to bring Tracy and Alison with us. Alison had done so much for Tracy – and for me – I wanted her to enjoy time there, too.

It was a substantial test for Tracy. To keep himself going on bad days, he clung to the image of himself sometime in the future acting like he had in the past. And we encouraged that picture every day. If he was ever going to be independent -- and live anything like he had in his former life -- he'd need to be able to fly and do everything that goes with that: getting on the plane with his baggage, finding his seat, knowing what to do if there was an emergency and locating the baggage claim and ground transportation. Earlier in the year, we had gone to places in Portland on MAX, our public transit light-rail system. We asked Tracy to tell us what our stop was for where we were going. He was able to tell us and he understood how to get where he wanted to go. Each time he met a milestone, it made me so grateful. I thought of him eighteen months before when he couldn't get out of his hospital bed and lived in a darkened and silent room tied down by all sorts of tubes with a Pink Pig close at hand in case he vomited.

And so, at the last of January 2013, we got ourselves to Portland International Airport on MAX and to the Hawaiian Airlines check-in counter and gate for our five-hour flight to Honolulu. Every step of the trip we offered Tracy choices. He chose to walk, not use a wheelchair, to get to the boarding gate. He also chose not to use the moving sidewalk, saying the people around him would not appreciate what he might do in reaction to the movement, and he hadn't brought his Pink Pig with him. I brought a more discreet vomit bag, just in case, but didn't tell him. I asked if he wanted to take advantage of early boarding. Early-on in this new life we were living, I learned that anytime I asked Tracy to make a decision, I found it best to ask Tracy well in advance of when the decision needed to be made. If he felt any pressure to hurry, or to make a quick decision, or just do something quckly and spontaneously, he fell apart. He'd stop in his tracks, become very agitated, grow angry and then refuse to do anything. Once I asked him what was going on when that happened, and he said it was as if someone poured something all over the top of him and he couldn't function. Being pressured by someone isn't pleasant any time, but under his circumstances, I wasn't going to do that to him. Alison also got it. Bill, however, didn't. If something is obvious to Bill, he assumes it's also obvious to everyone – and that they would agree with his conclusions because, of course, they were the right ones. Often that's the case, but not always. After my question about early boarding, Tracy verbally went through his decision tree. At each point when he paused, Bill would assume he was finished, and say, "That's it then. OK!" But Tracy wasn't finished. Both became frustrated. After Tracy decided that early boarding was a good idea for him so he didn't have to weave down a long aisle full of moving people on both sides of him as he tried to keep his balance, I asked Bill if he'd board right behind Tracy. In case Tracy fell, Bill would be the best one to help him right himself in such a confined space. Tracy struggled to be as independent as possible. Bill, in an effort to help, took his arm to steer him. Tracy resisted. Bill became annoyed. Wow, the trip was off to a terrific start!

We made it to the Hale Koa without much further angst. Tracy was testing to ascertain if he could be independent while still within view of people who could rescue him, if necessary. Bill, however, couldn't figure out what he was supposed to do to "be ready." So he wandered off. It worked out. Alison and I were enough to give Tracy reassurance without smothering him. Bill said Tracy was doing fine without him, so he wasn't going to worry about it. After settling in, Tracy took his camera with him and launched on an individual journey of his own.

The Hale Koa is a facility geared to people in all stages of life, including those with various physical limitations, so it was a perfect place for Tracy to wander around on his own for the first time in a year-and-a-half. He'd also been there before with us, and remembered the layout. My favorite picture that I hold in my heart of that trip is the smile on Tracy's face as he held his camera, standing on the sands of Waikiki Beach looking over the Pacific Ocean into the setting sun. Later he said the time at the Hale Koa was so special because for the first time in a very long while, he could go out by himself and be alone. For a person who values his own personal space and time, that was a giant gift. Our ten days in paradise went fast, but we made the most of each one.

Northwest Oregon often presents its residents a special weather gift: in mid-February, just when everyone has had it with cold, gray, rainy days, the temperature rises, the sun finds its way through the clouds for a day or two and everyone smiles and says, "Wow, I remember, this is what spring is like!"

I used that time to poke about in the garden, pruning roses and seeing where I could find early signs of life in the dirt. Tracy used it to just be outside. The first spring he was at our house in Beaverton, he sat in his wheelchair and graduated to small turns around the sidewalk and driveway using his walker and then his trekking pole. This spring, he started with his trekking pole. I can see him in my mind's eye leaning on his trekking pole, face to the sun. It was a sharp contrast to his being stiff as a tree trunk leaning against the corner in the kitchen when we first started having him stand up.

As the weeks passed, Tracy was itching to start walking in earnest. At first, he walked with one of us down the street and back; then down to Greenway Park and eventually along the Fanno Creek Trail in the park. He worked up to walking about a mile at this point. As he gained his footing and his confidence, he asked to go alone, taking his cell phone with him. He might have known it, but never spoke of my being behind him for the first few times he went "alone." I couldn't just let him go out of sight without reassuring myself that he would be O.K. He humored me, responding with our address when I asked him and telling me his planned route. I followed him the whole way for the first few times, then part of the way after that for a few more times, and then I took a deep breath and let him go. At the time, I thought it was just as hard to let go as it had been to "care" for him earlier when he was very limited in what he did.

I have heard opinions from some that bringing back an adult with a traumatic head injury must be similar to working with children. That opinion was usually from an outside perspective, and generally untrue. In some ways, yes, Tracy behaved like a child. He saw the world in clear unambiguous colors, no gray. Things were good or bad. Exercises were hard. He formed immediate opinions, had definite food dislikes and was not interested in changing his mind about them. He needed careful supervision but actively didn't like careful supervision, so it had to be done, well, carefully.

Adults are not children. Children have yet to have life experiences as reference points while adults retrieve memories that guide their decisions. Just because they may act like or seem like children in some parts of their behavior, doesn't mean they respond well to being treated as children. I found the biggest difference to be in the area of decision-making. Even though it took Tracy awhile to make a decision (not so unlike his Libra-like pre-stroke behavior), it was imperative that he be included in any decision relating to him – and if I didn't like the decision he made, I needed to figure out a way to live with it because Tracy is an adult, not a child. Tracy going for independent walks in Greenway Park was a decision he made that I lived with. It turned out to be another example of his good judgment.

A typical week for us included bridge for me on Monday; a pedicure for Tracy, Alison and me once a month on a Tuesday; speech clinic on Wednesdays; a massage every other week on Thursday – Cheryl continued to undo knots in Tracy's neck, shoulders and back; a doctor's visit and a trip to the dentist, a pharmacy run, and I had gone back to physical therapy twice a week for my shoulders and neck. Alison also went to physical therapy for her shoulder, but unfortunately, it was for too short a time for optimum recovery from her shoulder surgery. After we returned from Hawaii, I had cataract surgery because everything now looked gray, and I wasn't able to see well enough to drive at night. We had Tracy walking every day and continuing his daily speech and cognitive exercises. Bill continued to orchestrate plenty of symphonies, operas and ballets to attend on the weekends in his relished role as family social director.

In early spring 2013, I took a deep breath, and tackled Tracy's financial and tax situation.

Chapter 4:
Student Loans and the Fleecing of America

While going through Tracy's financial records soon after his stroke, I came upon the Tar Baby known as student loans. He had taken out a three-thousand-dollar student loan toward his bachelor's degree in 1982-83. Subsequently, he took out student loans toward his master's degree (a master of fine arts (MFA) in visual design with an emphasis in photography) totaling $29,000 over four years. An MFA is a "terminal" degree, comparable to a Ph.D. in other fields. Tracy assumed he would teach full-time at the college level and pay back his student loans fully and on-time.

For the next fourteen years, Tracy tried hard to reach his professional goal, a goal that had taken eight years of university education. He secured three adjunct (temporary) positions at three universities, and, although he subsequently made it to the final round in each case, he secured no permanent position. With the exception of one nine-week period, none of the temporary positions offered benefits, and all paid entry-level wages.

When he wasn't teaching, he worked to re-invent himself so he could make a living until he could find a teaching position. He continued photographing the world around him and filled in with seasonal spot work in construction and landscape design and installation to feed himself. He delved into book-making and crafting posters. He hosted and managed websites. He worked in retail selling glass art. His body of photographic work – mostly black and white – grew. While he knew that he was a good photographer, I think he had less self-confidence, early-on, as an oil-on-canvas artist, believing his niche was more teaching. Now his drive to produce art on canvas came to the fore. He began to experiment with oils and acrylics – usually bright colors – in large format.

During good times, Tracy made and sold many paintings that are hung all over the world. Economically, life was always a struggle. Tracy's life has never been one that included a regular paycheck sufficient to pay the bills. He lived simply. Once I heard him musing whether he might have been better off, *i.e.,* more successful, had he gone to the Art Institute of Chicago to become an artist rather than having attended the University of Oregon to become a college teacher.

Over time, Tracy made student-loan payments, but not on a scheduled basis, and there appeared to be a definite -- but unclear -- outstanding balance due on his student loans. I recall that Tracy and I talked about his frustration with the student-loan "thing" a few months prior to his stroke. At that time, I asked him if he had talked to someone about the whole mess. He said that, over the years, he had talked with student-loan representatives "hundreds of times." They always wanted a regular amount paid monthly and never understood why he found that impossible to do. At first, when he was attempting to teach, he tried to explain that, although he was teaching in his field, the position was a temporary one and he received a beginning level base pay with no benefits. One representative suggested that, since he was making an income below the poverty-level, he should accept welfare to pay back his student loans. Later, when he made his living as an artist, student-loan representatives never understood that he didn't receive a regular paycheck. They never understood the concept of being paid for completed work rather than for time spent on a job.

I asked how much he specifically owed. He said the answer wasn't as straight-forward as one might think. Over the years, he never received regular statements or invoices for his student loans. I have asked other people who had student loans if that was true. They said they always had trouble getting information, including principal and interest amounts, from either the Department of Education or private lenders. Although no student loan representative could break out the principle/interest figures of loan(s), they were very efficient at taking any tax refund he ever received. When Tracy asked for an accounting of how the amount ballooned from the original $29,000 loan to more than $98,000, no one could, or would, tell him how it happened. He just knew that they said he had seven loans to repay. He had taken out two loans that mysteriously multiplied into seven, or according to one representative, had been "re-packaged" into seven different loans. He could see no way out. For someone who lived on very little, $98,000 might just as well have been $98,000,000.

Was Tracy just a "bad apple" in the student loan barrel? Or was his situation indicative of a much larger problem?

According to the website, Debt.org, "Federal loans carry a six-month grace period so there is time to develop a plan for dealing with them. Most student borrowers, however, aren't that lucky. They leave with an average of $30,000 of debt and it is not unusual to owe that money to 8-10 separate lenders and potentially a combination of private and federal loans. Continuing on to graduate school can add another 4-6 lenders to the mix. Each one of these student loans has its own due dates, interest rates and payment amounts. Keeping track of that many payments is complicated... "

As reported in a January 2014 online article, 'Politicians Scramble to Fix Broken Student Loan System as Write-Offs Soar,' by Bill Fay, " ... The Consumer Financial Protection Bureau estimates that 7 million borrowers are in default, and that another 9 million have loan payments deferred or in forbearance, meaning they aren't making payments because they are in financial distress, unemployed, in the military or have re-enrolled in school. Those in deferral or forbearance are carrying about $212 billion of the estimated $1 trillion federal student loan debt. Private lenders are owed another $200 billion — bringing the total for student loan debt to $1.2 trillion."

For perspective, in 2015, according to the website, collegedebt.com, current student loan debt in the United States is more than $1.3 trillion; credit-card debt for the same period is $882 billion, and auto loan debt is $750 billion.

Clare McCann at New America wrote online in September, 2014 that the Department of Education reported a little more than one in five loans for undergraduate education will default within two decades.

Again according to Bill Fay in his January 2014 article, economists say the burden of student loans, combined with fewer job opportunities and lower salaries, are two reasons the economic recovery is slow. U.S. senators Dick Durbin, D-Ill., Jack Reed, D-R.I. and Elizabeth Warren, D-Mass introduced legislation in 2013 to address student-loan debt. Senator Warren stated, "Our higher education system is broken, and we need to make fixing it a real priority. We can start by restoring consumer protections to student loans, which are crushing our families."

How did this happen? How had higher education been hijacked? How had higher education gone from helping students and enriching American communities to becoming a racket to make money for financial institutions that issue student loans? It appears to me that financial assistance programs to benefit students were restructured to create a revenue stream for banker buddies of politicians who, in turn, receive big direct or indirect campaign contributions – all paid for on the backs of students.

I worked to piece together the student-loan information I found at Tracy's house in a file, his taxes, and some bills from mysterious companies such as ECSI and Premier Credit of North America, but, I confess, it was beyond me. I couldn't make heads-or-tails out of the paperwork. I couldn't figure out how many loans there were, the principal, interest, who owned the loan or the current amount due. But all of the various bills and other paperwork indicated the amount still owed was substantial. How in the world had this situation gotten so out of control?

I needed to get involved because Tracy's health precluded him from addressing his student loan situation for a substantial length of time, if ever. I knew how agitated he became when we discussed this situation well before his stroke. With doctors insisting that his life now must be as "stress-free" as possible, I had to handle this on my own. I wondered who might help me figure this out. I thought of Tracy's friend, Jane, who I knew had a debilitating disease and who had student loans. She said there was a very limited possibility that his loans might be forgiven because of his stroke. She encouraged me to find someone at the University of Oregon or the "national student-loan office" who might be able to help me resolve Tracy's student-loan debt. That brought me to a second person: Allen from the University of Oregon's financial aid office. His name appeared on lots of the paperwork in Tracy's student-loan file. I called him and asked if he recalled Tracy. He said he did. I told him what happened to Tracy. I asked him if he thought there was any way out of this mess. He told me there was indeed a possibility that Tracy's student loans might be forgiven based on illness and continued disability. He said that more loans were now being discharged due to "total and permanent disability." I later read that loans that have been discharged for this reason grew from fewer than 15,000 in 2008 to 115,700 in 2013. Allen told me there would be … forms to fill out. More forms.

The forms, titled "Discharge Application: Total and Permanent Disability," were from the U.S. Department of Education, and each loan required a separate completed form. I asked Allen how many loans there were and he said he thought there were nine or ten. Two were still held by the university and he promised he would move the discharge request for them to the right place. The rest were somewhere else. The forms required a physician's certification written directly on the form along with a letter on letterhead or a pharmacy pad signed by the doctor. The certification covered "Ability to Engage in Substantial Gainful Activity," "Disabling Condition," and "Limitations." I also attached a copy of the Power of Attorney to each form, which would allow me to act on Tracy's behalf. Without that, I could neither give nor receive information about him. One month after Tracy suffered his stroke, I sent that form to Allen at the University of Oregon and he forwarded copies to where they needed to go.

Based upon the fine print in the application, it seemed that once the U.S. Department of Education received the forms and their attendant documentation, the department would review the paperwork for completeness and send it on to the student-loan holder(s). Then the loan holder(s) would review the application and the documentation for completeness and determine whether it met their requirements for "totally and permanently disabled." Then the form(s) were returned to the Department of Education, which, in turn, reviewed the documentation to determine if the applicant was "totally and permanently disabled." After that, the applicant would be notified as to the outcome and whether they would enter a "discharge monitoring period" of three years from the date of the decision to determine if they were still "totally and permanently disabled." After a "successfully" completed monitoring period, the applicant's student loans would be forgiven. In a perverse way, it almost seemed as if making it through the monitoring period constituted a sort of accomplishment. How being totally and permanently disabled is somehow a success is beyond me.

As I delved into the murky world of student loans, I really felt as if I had tumbled down a rabbit hole. Nothing made sense. One eerily prescient note I found in Tracy's writing in his file, dated May 8, 2008, indicated he had told a student-loan representative that he was denying himself medical attention already because he couldn't earn enough to pay for it and student loans and still eat. I have no idea what medical problem concerned Tracy at that time.

How could there be nine or ten loans? He borrowed money for his two degrees, and even if the loans were issued one for each year, that was at most four or five loans. I discovered later that when loans were sent around different places within the U.S. Department of Education, as well as to outside private collection agencies that lurk in the shadows of the student-loan world, and other private finance institutions that bought delinquent loans, then the amount of the loan was jacked up by about 25 percent each time. They were sold, the loans were split, spliced, diced, repackaged and resold many times. Unpaid interest appeared to have been capitalized, not regularly but haphazardly. Each time, the loans were assigned a new number with new balances due, more fees and interest, another new representative, and the number of loans multiplied like rabbits.

The Internal Revenue Service and the Oregon Department of Revenue were involved periodically, too, in Tracy's student-loan fracas. In previous years, when Tracy filed his taxes and, if he were due a refund, the refund was sent instead to service his student loans. But, as I came to discover, none of the money sent to student-loan holders was credited to the actual principal outstanding amount. It was eaten up by interest, fees and "costs."

The process to discharge the loans is time-consuming, convoluted and confusing – not just to me but also to the loan holders because they continued to send dun notices. I called or emailed every company or agency that sent a notice. Every time I was told I couldn't talk to them about Tracy even though I had sent in the Power of Attorney information to the U.S. Department of Education. The company representatives said they knew nothing of any Power of Attorney.

Over the next few months, Allen, the University of Oregon student-loan officer, was a terrific help. If I didn't understand something, he was there to try to answer my questions. If something got lost, as in I sent it to the U.S. Department of Education and it disappeared, he helped me find it.

A little more than a week after I sent the paperwork to begin the "discharge" request process, another letter arrived, this time from the National Payment Center of the U.S. Department of Education. I was impressed. I thought, what an efficient response! I was disabused of any such notion when I opened the correspondence. I guess that since my request was sent through the University of Oregon to somewhere else, the folks at the National Payment Center in Georgia didn't know what the other hand was doing. Their letter indicated that yet another party, Diversified Collection Services, Inc. (DCS, Inc.) was commencing collection efforts on the full amount due. This was the first time I had seen what the student-loans folks said was the amount due on Tracy's loans. The principal balance outstanding was $39,873.22, which appeared to be about $10,000 more than what Tracy thought the original loan amount was, so, obviously, very little of Tracy's payments were applied toward the principal. "Interest" was listed at

$53,862.62 and "fees and costs" totaled $22,815.31. The total amount listed as now due was $116,551.15.

I looked at that form for a very long time. How on God's green earth was it legal for a loan of $32,000 to balloon into more than $116,000? And, how could Tracy ever pay it, especially now?

I called the number listed in the letter. I spoke with someone, explaining that Tracy had a stroke. The person I spoke with said he was not allowed to speak to me about Tracy because he had not seen a Power of Attorney. But, he also said he was authorized to accept a credit card number that very minute to pay the bill in full! Failing that, he said, he could discuss a payment plan or repayment program with either Tracy or me. I explained that Tracy was unable to discuss this or anything else at this time. After a momentary pause, the man said, "Well, you could just give us your credit-card number." I declined to do that. Like most people's credit cards, my credit card isn't designed to accept a one-time $116,000 smack on it. Besides, I was helping Tracy to the extent I could, but paying old loans to people I didn't know for an amount I couldn't believe was legitimate, wasn't going to be part of my help.

A week after that, Tracy received a letter from the University of Oregon stating that based on their review of my application for Tracy for Total and Permanent Disability Discharge, they were assigning his file to the U.S. Department of Education for review. The letter went on to state that the Department of Education would make an initial determination for discharge and would request income information during the "conditional" period. Also, the letter instructed us not to make any payments unless specifically instructed to do so by the Department of Education. (Did that mean the fellow from Diversified Collection Services, Inc. was acting on the Department of Education's behalf or just taking a flying leap on his own?) Finally, as in all future correspondence and discussions I had on this issue, the letter indicated that if the Department of Education determined that Tracy wasn't eligible for a "Total and Permanent Disability Discharge," they would notify us and collection activities would again begin on the account.

In a letter dated September 20, 2011, the U.S. Department of Education "Total and Permanent Disability Servicer" indicated that they now would be servicing his loan and that they would be assisting the Department of Education in the "application review" process. The letter gave lots of contact information, including a correspondence address in Denver, Colorado.

There were two problems with this letter, as I saw it. First, they weren't using Tracy's correct name, although I had given it to them, and second, I received this letter at the end of the next March, more than six months after it was written. By the way, they never got Tracy's name right.

I received a four-page letter dated March 2, 2012, (and received April 30, 2012), from an organization calling itself "nelnet." "Nelnet's" letterhead included in its listing "Education Planning & Financing" and identified itself as the U.S. Department of Education's "Total and Permanent Disability Servicer." In the letter, "nelnet" wrote that it had completed its review of Tracy's application for a total and permanent disability discharge. The department had discharged his loan or service obligation on the basis of his total and permanent disability. I felt a surge of joy that this burden was being lifted from a pair of shoulders that would never be able to carry such a load. I continued reading the letter.

In the first paragraph, the letter listed several loans, all with long names and separate acronyms, most of which I had never heard of. The list appeared to include all the types of loans he might have, but hadn't necessarily, taken out. It also included a "service obligation," as well. It would help a lot if I could just figure out what, precisely, the loans were, what the service obligation was, and if this discharge covered all of them. Were there any others I hadn't yet discovered? I continued reading the letter.

Finally, on page four I found information seemingly tailored to Tracy, not just general boilerplate gobbledegook. At the top of the page was "Discharged Loan or TEACH Grant Service Obligation." The first item under that heading was one "TEACH Grant service obligation." Hooray! One Down! But then my hopes tumbled: Under the next heading, "Other Potentially Eligible Loan Information," the letter said that during their review of his application, "nelnet" had identified another loan that might be eligible for loan discharge based on his total and permanent disability, but to be considered, he must submit a total and permanent disability discharge application to the loan holder. I was getting dizzy again. We already had submitted those applications months ago to the U.S. Department of Education. If it wasn't the Department of Education, I didn't know who the loan holder(s) was. No one seemed to have a complete list.

After this paragraph was a list of ten loans that they said might be eligible for discharge. Nine of them were the same loan type. All had listed next to them "Loan ID," and "Holder." I grabbed Tracy's file. Now maybe we were getting somewhere. If I could match anything – Loan ID numbers or Loan Holders – I could see if this was a complete list. No numbers matched anything anywhere. Most of the "Holders" had N/A listed after them. Who were they? Mystery banks or secret collection agencies? I still don't know who those mystery/secret entities are, but "nelnet" seems to be yet another private company formed to make money on the backs of people snared by student loans. I will say that I could access their website and get helpful information, which was a first.

Finally, the letter reiterated that the loan(s) or "TEACH Grant service obligation(s)" had been discharged but that they would be reinstated if certain requirements during the three-year post-discharge monitoring period were not met. That seemed fair to me. I wasn't sure what the "post-discharge monitoring requirements" were, but surely we could meet them.

Having received the September letter at the end of March and the March letter at the end of April, I contacted Allen at the University of Oregon again, admitting I was confused. Based on the copies of the letters I provided to him, he was pretty confused, too. ESCI kept sending bills in the amount of $3,455.89 – an amount that made little sense given the total outstanding amount. Allen and I gave up trying to tease out which of the ten outstanding loans listed by the Department of Education in its March 2 letter actually applied to the University of Oregon loan. He said he'd do some research and get back to me. When he did, he said he'd had to wait over seven minutes to speak to someone about the status of Tracy's application for discharge, and that they had told him Tracy's request was being *reviewed*. That was May 7. I had a letter dated March 2 that said his application had been approved. I'm dizzy again. Allen's suggestion was that I wait until the dust settled to ascertain whether any more loans were out there to worry about. We both figured they'd be trying to contact Tracy if they still wanted money.

On May 23, 2012, I opened a letter to Tracy from yet another mystery financial institution, Financial Asset Management Systems, Inc, aka FAMS. Their opening salvo was that his defaulted student loans had been placed with FAMS for the purpose of "securing payment of this debt." Hmmm. The previous September letter (that showed up in March) from the U.S. Department of Education had stated that it would service Tracy's loan or service obligation "from this point forward." I assumed that to mean from the date of their letter, which preceded the FAMS letter by eight months and three days. This outfit said he owed a different amount: $120,251.59. Of course, they kept adding on interest, fees and "costs," so of course the total due would keep rising. In their letter, they offered several clever and fast ways in which to pay the amount they wanted to collect. If we wanted to pay by phone, we could call a toll-free number or go on their website and scan a Quick Response Code to have the money removed immediately from a bank account.

I called the contact phone number in the letter. I was encouraged to pay the amount they said was owed. I declined. However, I got to speak with a live representative in their Debt Management and Collections Office, where they handled what they called "Default Resolutions." During our discussion, I asked if they had a list of Tracy's outstanding loans. Helpfully, they did. They also provided me an address for the U.S. Department of Education so I was able to get the latest information from them. The address was in Greenville, Texas, not Georgia or Denver, Colorado. I asked that they refrain from sending further dunning letters to Tracy since the U.S. Department of Education was considering discharge of his loan due to total and permanent disability. They agreed and kept their word.

In October, 2012, I wrote the U.S. Department of Education at the Greenville, Texas, address, since that was the last one I'd received for them. I asked several questions to clarify that the loans listed in their March 2 letter were indeed the total number of loans outstanding. I had waited for the dust to settle, as Allen suggested, but I concluded that seven months was long enough.

In November, 2012, I received a letter from "nelnet" saying exactly the same thing that was included in the September, 2011 letter more than a year ago – it was an exact copy. The correspondence address was back in Denver, not Greenville, Texas, though, so maybe that was the problem. Denver and Greenville weren't sharing information, and I don't know whatever happened to Georgia. Thus, we were back to being told that they had received Tracy's application and were looking at it. There was no mention of the letter in between which said his application was approved and he was entering a three-year post-discharge monitoring period. Nor were my questions answered about the total number of outstanding loans.

On January 24, 2013, we received a letter from "nelnet" requiring submission of documentation of Tracy's employment income for 2012 by March 25, 2013. I understood the purpose of this submission was to meet requirements to continue the disability discharge application during the three-year monitoring period which Tracy apparently had entered, but to me, the timing was odd. I asked if I could send them information after I had completed doing Tracy's taxes and their answer was that they expected to receive the "proof of employment income" information for the previous year on the anniversary date of the start of the three-year monitoring period which is January 19, 2012. That was the first time I saw the January 19 date.

In February, 2013, I emailed a letter to "nelnet." I wrote that in January, 2013, we received a 1099-C, Cancellation of Debt, stating that $6,759 of loan debt had been discharged. Where did that amount come from? Was it part of one of the loans we knew about or part of another loan? I again called Allen at the University of Oregon. He could make no sense of the amount and he's a student-aid professional.

I concluded my February, 2013 letter to "nelnet" with another list of questions, more than one of which, I admit, was a bit snarky. But I was getting annoyed. My questions included:

Did you receive my letter of October 24, 2012? In it I detailed several loans. Have they been rolled-up into one?

Are there other loans not included for some reason even though our application was for total and permanent disability discharge of ALL of Tracy's student loans?

Where does the $3,455.89 fit in?

If you did receive my letter, when are you going to answer it?

Where did the discharge of $6,759 come from? Is it part of the loans in the discharge application? If so, why was it discharged and not the others?

I was astonished to receive an email response in two days. The responder indicated that they had received my October letter, but "unfortunately, it is not part of our process to respond to mailed correspondence unless it is critical to the discharge of the borrowers' loans currently in our system." OK, I guess institutional rudeness is the norm these days. Importantly, though, they did answer that they had all of Tracy's loans. No other shoe was waiting to drop. There appeared to be no rationale for discharging the debt of $6,759 in 2012. I guess it was just the first one they landed on. I shuddered when I thought of the remaining amount waiting to be discharged/cancelled. A 1099 was a direct attention-getter to the Internal Revenue Service. I figured I'd know how bad the tax was when I finished Tracy's taxes for the year. As to the $3,445.89, who knows? Again in fairness, the responder was polite and included a way to reach him/her (their title in the email was "TPD

Servicing") should I have further questions.

Sadly, we weren't finished with garbled correspondence. I sent the requested "proof of employment income" information for the previous year, along with completed income tax forms to the address "nelnet" provided (the Denver address) on March 1. On March 25, a letter arrived threatening reinstatement of his student loans if we didn't send "proof of employment income information for the previous year" by May 24. On April 2, I responded that we had indeed sent it and I was concerned identity theft was a real possibility if they didn't know where that tax information was located. On April 5, I received an email stating that they had received the information on March 13, processed it on April 4, and all was O.K. for another year.

The discharge-monitoring period was three years: January 19, 2012-2015. Each January, I sent proof of employment income information for the previous year. To date, Tracy has nowhere near exceeded the employment-income guidelines to remain eligible. In 2012, one loan was discharged in the amount of $6,759. As with much else relating to student loans, I have no clue where they came up with that amount, but it more than doubled his taxable income for the year. Tax-wise, he went from a small refund to owing almost $1,000.

According to a March, 2014 *New York Times* article, "Disabled Borrowers Trade Loan Debt for a Tax Bill from the I.R.S.," "... After much criticism, the Department of Education has made it easier in recent years for disabled borrowers to have their federal student loans discharged. But now, as more people are qualifying for loan forgiveness, many of them are running into an unexpected consequence: They are often shocked to learn that they basically exchanged one debt for another ... Under current tax law, the amount of debt forgiven is generally taxable, so some disabled borrowers end up with tax bills they cannot afford ... "

In 2013, it got much worse. On May 6, the remaining loans were discharged in the amount of $98,347.53. Of that, $58,474.31 was considered interest. Instead of a small refund on his taxable income, Tracy faced a tax bill of almost $29,000. I have no idea where the sum of $98,347.53 came from nor how the amount of $58,474.31 was determined as interest. The 1099-C Cancellation of Debt, which announced this new development, indicated that the 1099-C was issued "by agreement" -- the capital letter 'F' in Box 6 – "Identifiable Event Code."

According to the IRS fine print, I subsequently found, the cancellation was the result of an agreement between creditor and debtor to cancel debt at less than full consideration. What agreement? How did "they" come up with the total amount and the amount of interest? Did asking for discharge because Tracy is totally and permanently disabled constitute an "agreement?" As to the amount, again, I have no idea how it was determined. It matches no paperwork I have seen. I also was unclear as to the timing of the discharge. Tracy remained in a monitoring period until January, 2015, before student-loan officials consider this debt officially cancelled. So how is it that he is expected to pay income tax on the discharge of a loan that wouldn't officially be completed for another nineteen months? What would happen if, God forbid, "they" decided to "un-cancel" the discharge of his student-loan debt?

At this point there was another trip down the rabbit hole. Once a student-loan debt is cancelled or discharged, the IRS considers it income. If a creditor has discharged a debt a person owes, that person is required to include the discharged amount in their reported income. Surely, I thought, there must be some exception to this. It wasn't as if Tracy decided to have a stroke to renege on paying student loans. As Tax Day loomed, I was in a state of absolute dismay. While my brother had made amazing progress from his massive stroke almost three years ago, it has forever changed him and his life. It's astonishing that he's alive. Each day is a struggle and a challenge for him. He is not well enough – nor capable enough -- to work. How is he supposed to pay a tax bill of $29,000? When Tracy saw the 1099, he was confused. When I said it related to student loans and I attempted to simply explain how student loans had turned into income, he became highly agitated. Tracy doesn't need many things, and one thing he absolutely doesn't need is stress that elevates his blood pressure. I told him it was my worry to deal with, not his.

After completing Tracy's taxes in two forms, one without the student loan cancellation of debt and one that included it, I worked out how to talk to the IRS and the Oregon Department of Revenue about resolution of this gargantuan and ridiculous issue. First, I checked both the IRS and the Oregon Department of Revenue websites to see how to contact my local offices to make appointments with agents. On the face of it that seemed to me a reasonable approach. How silly of me. As far as the IRS is concerned, they don't take phone calls or schedule appointments with "regular" people, like me. I'm sure if I were a high-powered tax attorney, I'd be able to secure an appointment. I also bet I'd be able to get through the security gauntlet at my local IRS office without having to take off my boots and walk through the trail of mud left on the floor by previous visitors.

As far as the Oregon Department of Revenue is concerned, I waited forty-five minutes on the phone before I talked with a man who sounded pretty bored. I admit, if I had his job, I'd probably not be happy either. First, he told me he had no clue why the receptionist connected me to his phone number because he was in the debt-collection department and didn't answer tax-law questions. I told him I thought I had a debt-collection question but he disagreed. And, anyway, he couldn't talk to me unless I had authorization to speak on behalf of my brother. When I told him that the reason I was calling was to learn how to get that authorization, he walked me through where to find the proper form online. He told me that I should just file Tracy's taxes on time without paying the tax bill and wait to hear from the State's bill collectors.

I checked further on the IRS website to see if I could figure out what form I needed for authorization to represent Tracy. It goes without saying that government agencies like their own authorization forms. They don't use Power of Attorney forms accepted by everyone else. I found Form 2848 "Power of Attorney and Declaration of Representative," and then tried to find what I could relating to "student-loan debt" and "cancellation of debt." There are many forms and publications that at first glance seem to relate to this subject, but mostly they relate to bankruptcy or "principal-residence indebtedness," business or corporate debt, farm indebtedness, or credit-card debt, not student loans.

When I couldn't get the help I needed from the government agencies that are funded via my tax dollars to service me and other citizens, I turned to an even better source of wisdom: my Bridge Sisters. We'd been playing bridge together every Monday for the last few years, and it never ceases to amaze me what a broad array of knowledge emanates from that group. One "sister" had a daughter-in-law who worked in the legal/advocacy section of the IRS. Another had a son in law school, who was volunteering at a Lewis and Clark College law clinic open to the public. Each reached out for me. We discovered that the local the IRS office no longer offered legal advice and assistance to taxpayers. (About the same time, my Bridge Sister told me her daughter-in-law had just been transferred to another division.) I held the information regarding the tax clinic in case I couldn't get a response from the IRS. I was concerned that the issue I was trying to resolve was so esoteric that it would be beyond law students at a public clinic, although I was pretty sure they would be interested and want to help.

I contacted my U.S. Representative's office to see who they might suggest I call to find how to see a live person at the IRS. I thought I would need a live person to show them my completed Form 2848, "Power of Attorney and Declaration of Representative" which Tracy had signed. If I didn't see someone in-person, how could they see the authorization form? Sure enough, Joyce who is my U.S. Representative's in-house expert on all things related to taxes, gave me a phone number for the Taxpayer Advocates Office. (My U.S. Representative's staff person expressed astonishment when I told her that cancelled student loans are considered income.)

I called the local number of the Taxpayer Advocates Office and got a recording, so I called the national number and talked with the man who answered the telephone. I explained my situation and was told to take the problem, along with all appropriate paperwork, to my local IRS office and talk with an agent. He said that the IRS needed to determine if "this" was a "taxable event," and, if so, whether it was collectable or not. He said if the IRS determined it wasn't collectable this year, they would likely just keep collecting interest on the debt and take another look next year and probably for the next ten years before they decided maybe they'd write it off. Ten years?

Two days later, I hopped on a MAX train, our area's light-rail system, a little after 8 a.m. and traveled to the IRS office in Portland. That's where I got to take my boots off. After I got my boots back on and everything back into my pockets and my bag, I asked how to find the IRS. A security guard pointed past a bank of elevators, and said, "Turn left and go down the stairs." I rounded the corner, found the top of the stairs, and descended the steps to Hell.

The whole place was lifeless and deathly quiet. The wide spiral staircase dumped out into a long dark corridor enclosed on one side by dark glass. Several human forms moved like silent ghosts behind the glass. At the far end was a cubicle of glass in which stood a woman bathed in light behind a chest-high counter. The sign on the door announced WAIT HERE. I did. She waved me in and asked what I needed. I explained I needed to see an agent about my brother's tax issue relating to cancellation of a student loan. She said, "Oh, we don't offer live assistance on tax law issues anymore in this office. You'll have to call and talk with someone on the phone, or you can go to the website."

My friends all laugh at the poker face I do not have. Everything, I guess, is reflected on my face. In my head, I saw several cartoon figures lying motionless on a floor, offering "dead assistance." I tried to be polite. I asked how I could use either my phone or my computer since I had the physical piece of paper for the Power of Attorney in my possession. It would do little good to show it to my phone or my computer. She said she'd fax it for me. So, my trip was worthwhile. She said it would be about ten days to two weeks before it got into the system and attached to Tracy's tax file. Now I was looking at somehow resolving this after April 1. Tax Day was getting closer.

The IRS woman gave me the "special" phone number to use when I called asking for help on this issue. I looked at it: 1-800-829-1040. It's the same number everyone calls for personal income tax information. I already had waited on that line for many minutes before and never got into the system. I discovered "they" automatically kicked you off the system after twenty-five minutes and I had to start over. But, she gave me the name of the publication and the form required to move on. She suggested I try next door in the File Room and see if they had copies. They didn't have a copy of the publication (not very commonly requested they said) but they thought they had the form in the "Back Room." I waited. A few minutes later, I got the answer: sorry, not there after all. But their faces brightened, I could download it from their website. I returned home and jumped on my computer to get Publication 4681, "Cancelled Debts, Foreclosures, Repossessions, and Abandonments (for Individuals)" because that was the form I was told handled our situation. It didn't look too promising by the title, but I began reading. I read all twenty-five pages of the publication. Student loans were mentioned on page four under "Exceptions," but it related to people who worked for a certain period of time in the teaching profession after college and thus didn't pertain to Tracy's particular situation, so I read on. There was nothing else in the publication dealing directly with student-loan cancellation. I delved deep into "exceptions and exclusions" to the general rule that a canceled debt is included in income to determine whether anything suited Tracy's situation. I found nothing written that specifically addressed cancellation of student-loan debt. I slogged through more verbiage.

Finding nothing germane in Publication 4681, I made the leap to "insolvency," "recourse debt," the insolvency worksheet and reporting insolvency on Form 982 "Reduction of Tax Attributes Due to Discharge of Indebtedness." None of the several examples given in the publication covered student loans. The closest example was of a credit-card debt in "insolvency more than canceled debt."

In the March, 2014 *New York Times* article, "Disabled Borrowers Trade Loan Debt for a Tax Bill from the I.R.S.," the article notes, "…Borrowers who can prove they are insolvent may be able to ease the tax burden…and many people do not even know this exception exists. The insolvency calculation is notoriously complex…" Boy, howdy, was that on target!

I concluded that the only solution that suited Tracy's situation was insolvency. He had no assets; he didn't own a home; his vehicle had 'way more than one-hundred-thousand miles on it. I'd whittled down his bills, but there were several still lurking in the background. I pulled together the information to complete the insolvency worksheet.

The lady at the IRS told me to pay attention to the Date of Identifiable Event on the 1099-C. Now I knew why. I had to put together a picture of Tracy's financial situation on the day *before* the day the loan (a liability) was cancelled and it turned into income (an asset). Adding the student-loan debt to his other debts certainly exceeded his assets. One is considered insolvent if their liabilities exceed their assets. After I gathered all the information and checked what he owned and owed, I completed the worksheet. I turned to Form 982 as Publication 4681 instructed. In Part I, I was to check Line 1b "Discharge of indebtedness to the extent insolvent (not a title 11 case)" to report Tracy's insolvency. Also in Part I, I was to enter the "total amount of discharged indebtedness excluded from gross income on line 2." I entered the total amount of the student loan on the 1099-C. So far, so good, but there were two more Parts to go.

Part II stated: "Reduction of Tax Attributes. You must attach a description of any transactions resulting in the reduction in basis under section 1017. See Regulations section 1.1017-1 for basis reduction ordering rules, and, if applicable, required partnership consent statements (For additional information, see the instructions for Part II.)" I read all thirteen lines under Part II, which were headed "Enter amount excluded from gross income." I shook my head to clear it. I then turned to the instructions for Part II. I couldn't see how any of this related to Tracy's student loans. Maybe line 5 or 10a pertained? I had no clue. I could make no sense of what I had read. I put it aside and read it again the next day. It still made no sense. I attempted to reach the IRS again since I had whittled down my questions to just a couple. I checked the website once more for any help and decided to try the local Taxpayer Advocate Service again to find a local Taxpayer Advocate (called an LTA by the IRS).

I called. A man answered. I briefly described my reason for calling. I was getting good at being brief on this subject. I had a great deal of recent practice. He responded, "We don't do THAT, here! You need to go to a professional tax accountant or attorney, or if you are poor, I can give you the names and phone numbers of three groups that can help you. You can also try the VITA volunteers who help people file their taxes, as long as his tax forms don't include Schedule C, D, E, or F." Tracy's included a Schedule C, so that would't work. I'd served as a VITA volunteer years before in Alabama when Bill, my husband, was on active duty with the U.S. Army. Knowing the "training" I'd received to volunteer, I didn't hold out much hope that one of these well-meaning people would be able to help.

Since I was looking at declaring insolvency for my brother, it seemed obvious that he'd qualify for the "free" services just described. First, I called Catholic Charities and got a recording. Next, I called Legal Services of Oregon. I launched into my brief explanation … again. A woman told me they didn't handle things like that. She asked which county we lived in. I said I was in Washington County, but my brother lived in Lincoln County. She said I should call Lincoln County. I said I was acting on his behalf. She sounded pretty bored with the whole conversation, but said I could try the Washington County Legal Aid Office and gave me the phone number.

I called. The woman who answered also sounded bored (is that a requirement for those who answer phones?) and said they didn't do taxes or give tax advice, nor did they have any expertise in that area. I must to talk to an attorney.

I called the third group, Lewis and Clark College Legal Clinic… the same one I was holding in reserve from one of my Bridge Sisters. The woman who answered said it was a teaching clinic, worked by appointment only and didn't give out tax advice over the phone. She also said they didn't assist with filing taxes and would get involved if the "project" I brought them would take no more than three months to resolve and would be interesting to the students. Well, I certainly hoped the "project" would take no more than three months, but when I asked if she thought it could be resolved prior to April 15 of this year, she said, "Oh, absolutely not." She did suggest that if we had further difficulties later with the IRS, I could request assistance then because it might be more interesting. I had the feeling of somehow being stared at under a microscope while talking on the phone.

The same *New York Times* article, "Disabled Borrowers Trade Loan Debt for a Tax Bill from the I.R.S.," continues, "... People who find themselves with large tax obligations have to evaluate how to navigate the process on their own or with professional help, which can be hard to find. The IRS's free tax preparation service for low- and moderate-income people is not equipped to handle the complexities." I could now attest to all of the above.

I was back at square one.

I decided that if the IRS would not let me come to them, I'd complete Tracy's taxes as best I could and wait for them to come to me.

I went back into Turbo Tax, which I was using to do Tracy's taxes. Since he'd not used a Form 982 before, I couldn't figure how to get a new blank form to use now, so I pushed the Help Button at the top of my screen. In the space of less than two hours, I was provided answers by an accredited tax expert who said what I had been trying to do was correct. She helped me find Form 982 and a student-loan cancellation of debt/insolvency worksheet. She said I was good to go if there were no highlighted areas left on the form or worksheet and no red circled exclamation point next to the form in the list to the left of my computer screen, and no errors listed after I completed the taxes.

Are we finished with this episode? I hope so. I learned a lot about what not to expect from the IRS and the ancillary organizations that stay afloat inferring assistance but providing no help. I got a truck load of unwanted surprises along the way. However, I received never-wavering help and support, ideas, and suggestions from my friends when there were days I was so frustrated I was babbling.

I was left with one final question: How can regular people be expected to do all this? And what happens to someone like Tracy, if they don't?

Chapter 5:
A Walk in the Park:
Pictures and an iPhone Camera

Spring, 2013 progressed in its usual fits and starts. On our weekly trips to see Daria at the Legacy/Meridian Speech Clinic, a drive down Interstate 5 from our house, we walked through a little courtyard garden on the way to the meeting room. It was a great success at its purpose: offering calm and quiet reflection for patients, families and caregivers. The garden must help staff to slow down and take a breath as well. Someone who knew what they were doing created this garden. It is reflective of the seasons and has the sound of a fountain and a pleasing fragrance along with visual beauty. I noticed Tracy paid attention to it. He did something similar with the garden at our house. Over time, his vision improved, and now he was examining in depth ... leaf and rain patterns on the sidewalk. It made my heart happy. He hadn't lost his quirky way of examining the world!

A few days later, he asked where his iPhone was. We had kept it, but up to now it wasn't useful to him based on his limitations of sight and finger dexterity. Instead, we had gotten him a little "old person" phone with just the basics in big letters and numbers that he carried with him. Time marches on and heals, so I dug out his iPhone. By Apple standards, it was now ancient. It was time for an adventure to the Apple Store in our local shopping mall.

First, though, I brought up the Apple Store online so Tracy could examine their wares. He was entranced with the latest iPhone, and an updated iPad.

After that, he began to look more at his computer. He had made a tentative exploration of his earlier life on his computer some months earlier, and now it was like the floodgates opened. He spent hours looking at his paintings and photos online. Tracy still had difficulty fingering the keyboard so he wasn't interested in using it for email or to respond to Facebook messsages, but he did look at them.

We made an appointment at the Apple Store. Tracy had definite ideas about what he wanted and needed. He participated in a full and thorough discussion with the customer-service representative. Tracy came away from the Apple Store with a new iPhone, and shortly thereafter a newly refurbished iPad made its way into our house. He found the iPad easier to use than his computer, and spent time every day doing various brain exercises on it. The iPhone became his inseparable companion whenever he left the house. But, he actually wanted it for the camera, not to talk on it.

Near the last of March, on a glorious day, we had our third annual Honey Bee Swarm. I marvel that even though we live in suburbia, wildlife seems to find my garden. After seeing the weight of the large mass of bees dragging down one of the branches on my little Hemlock tree and then taking off on the next leg of their journey to find a new home only to come crashing down in the middle of the street, I put out Tracy's two orange "gelato" cones to warn traffic and called a beekeeper I found in the online Yellow Pages. He couldn't come until the next morning. I told him hundreds of bees were being run over and they'd all be dead if we waited another day. He said they were docile in a swarm so I should get a dust pan and brush, gently sweeping them up to deposit them in a safer place. I dutifully went out to rescue the bees. Is anyone laughing yet? I knew I wanted to bring them just a small distance from the middle of the street to underneath our Japanese maple tree at the edge of the sidewalk.

I began by gently sweeping up a few hundred of the many bees that were on the pavement. Someone forgot to tell the bees what was going on. They attacked. I felt them all over my face, ears, eyes, neck and hands. Luckily, I had on a long-sleeved shirt. I persevered because I figured I already was stung. After two dustpans full, I picked up the two cones, which were totally covered inside-and-out with bees. Later we discovered that the queen was in one of them. I put them under the tree and at that point frantically brushed off the bees still on me – and stinging.

I ran to the front door. Tracy was just inside the storm door, watching the entire episode. It must have looked hysterical: his sister gone mad, running in-and-out of the street with orange cones and a dustpan and brush, waving her hands frantically around her head in between trips to the street. Most of the bees did not pursue me. They were focused on protecting their queen. They were not seeking revenge. I asked Tracy to come outside to make sure there were no bees on me before I came into the house. Once in the house, I called Bill and our good friend and neighbor, Linda, but neither answered.

I asked Tracy to stay in the house and told him I was driving myself to our neighborhood Urgent Care, an emergency room of sorts, before my eyes swelled shut and I couldn't see. At Urgent Care I discovered it really could be urgent care if someone like me showed up with a bunch of bee stings. I was quickly stripped and two bees were found still alive inside my shirt. The physician's assistant and nurse pulled out nineteen stingers and found thirty bee stings. We waited to be sure I had no anaphylactic reaction.

Bill showed up at Urgent Care and took me home. We came back later and retrieved my car. Tracy was very concerned (probably more for my mental state (!) than for my physical distress) and I got royal treatment all afternoon from Bill and Tracy.

An interesting side note: all my various aching arthritic joints quit aching for several weeks after the bee stings. I'd heard of bee venom treatments and it looked like they worked for me!

Now for the rest of the story: we became friends with a honey of a beekeeper, who not only came to rescue the remaining bees (he estimated about fifteen-thousand of them) but he entertained and educated the neighbors about bees, while he gathered them up into a portable hive. He left another portable hive under our Japanese maple tree in case additional swarms arrived on the scene, which they did. But they went high up into the oak tree, where they were safe and able to rest. The beekeeper told me the reason the bees landed in the middle of the street was that they had an old queen who collapsed and couldn't go any farther. She crash-landed, and her bee escorts are programmed to stay with her and protect her. Hence, when she went down, they did, too. He surmised they took me as a predator because I cast a shadow over them when I attempted to pick them up.

Wildlife adventures continued in my garden. Later in June, Tracy watched the Great Finch Hatching, and, in the course of time, he helped in the garden during the day after their fledging, watching for predators until the birds could fly.

In early April 2013, I requested a referral from Tracy's doctor for another vestibular evaluation at Oregon Health Sciences University (OHSU). It was more than a year since the last referral, so we started the game over again. If I had asked for an earlier appointment from CareOregon with Andy, the OHSU physical therapist/vestibular guru, I wouldn't have gotten it. They were convinced Tracy had stabilized in a "current chronic condition" and, therefore, it was a waste of time to do anything for him in terms of therapy.

Tracy saw Andy for visits in April, May and June. Although Andy had requested more visits for him, CareOregon denied them. In those visits, they worked on several tasks including agility.

Tracy is a Scot by heritage. There's a sword dance they do using crossed swords on the ground. Tracy used crossed brooms on the floor, but I could hear the bagpipes reeling as he "danced" over, sideways, backwards and forwards around the brooms. I asked if he could hear them, and he laughed. Laughter helped as he tipped over and practiced his "three-point stance" for balance around the brooms.

Andy introduced Tracy to Tai Chi, saying it was something he could continue independently with a video. The other big things they did during those visits was evaluate whether he could handle the recumbent bike (a bicycle that places the rider in a laid-back reclining position in which the rider's weight is distributed more comfortably over a larger area), upper-body ergometer and treadmill. They calibrated speed, difficulty and time. Andy taught Tracy how to evaluate his exertion level since she did not want him getting exhausted, but she wanted him to progress.

She was satisfied with how he handled both the instructions (he was now able to comprehend and remember instructions in his short-term memory bank unlike earlier) and that he understood the purpose of the various exercises.

Andy explained to Tracy how to calculate pulse/exercise ratio. The treadmill was uniquely interesting in that she had him do side steps and turns at slower speeds by stepping off and on the treadmill while it was still moving. She said this helped train his vestibular system, and negotiating the turns with rails to hold on to made it safe for him.

One entertaining but difficult exercise she had Tracy do was skipping, using his fingertips along the wall for stability. Andy said he should work toward skipping without touching the wall with his fingers.

In response to the April visit, Tracy took considerable time, but he crafted an email to Andy, thanking her for her time, and asking "... I wanted to make sure that given my strokes that brought me into your wonderful care, that I have your blessing if I wanted to continue the gym-like workout. I am not talking winded, vigorous work-outs, but more than I have been doing? What are your thoughts? ... It was wonderful seeing you! And I have added you (sic) email to my computer, and you are welcome to add mine to yours. Wendy is my cc to make sure I have added the correct things -- and spelling! Sincerely, Tracy"

After another doctor's visit and completing all the proper forms, Tracy had an appointment for a personal-fitness interview with a trainer at our local Tualatin Hills Park & Recreation District's (THPRD) Elsie Stuhr Center. In early June, two months after starting this process, Tracy had his own identification card and approval to participate in activities at the fitness center. At his June appointment with Andy, he took with him a copy of the workout program he and the fitness trainer had designed. So much for his being "unable to benefit from further therapy at this time due his age and chronic condition."

During this time, I also asked Tracy's doctor for a referral to OHSU's occupational therapist (more than a year had passed since his last appointment with her) because Tracy and I were curious to see what changes had occurred that might bring him closer to driving a car again. Previously, Tracy was tested on a large machine with lights that went on-and-off. He was directed to hit a button when the light came on. He'd done poorly. Too much eye and body motion exhausted and nauseated him. He also wasn't able to see lights in the lower right quadrant of his vision. But, Tracy wanted to try it again.

He saw Amy, the OHSU occupational therapist, twice and was tested and retested on the machine. He did better, but was so deliberative about being right, he couldn't match the speed necessary. Amy said he showed improvement, but he still had a ways to go. Tracy's vision was improved; he didn't throw up. But, he concluded it wasn't imperative that he drive right away. That conclusion was very different from the last time he had taken this test. Then he clenched his teeth because he so desired to "pass" the exam so he could drive. Driving meant independence to him. It served as a mental talisman of "being well" like he was "before." I marveled at what a year had brought. He no longer desperately needed to drive to prove his "independence." He found *that* satisfaction now in other ways. He walked, texted and emailed; interacted with his friends; watched TV; talked with neighbors. He no longer was isolated in his little world. He could get out on his own without driving. I took him to see his SUV, Luna, which was still at my son's house. Tracy sat in the driver's seat, saying that it felt great. But as he climbed out of his SUV, he said, "Until I know I won't make a mistake that hurts someone else, I don't want to drive."

Spring 2013 brought company from cousins Mark and Kathy, who live in New Hampshire. They were so relieved at how they found Tracy. Facebook has been an immediate and efficient means of keeping folks informed, but sitting down and talking with Tracy in person, and seeing his reactions in real time, is so much more satisfying. The cousins invited Tracy to visit them in the fall. It was interesting to watch his reaction. The suggestion was one he had not considered, and now someone had said it out loud, making it in the realm of possibility. He took hold of it and for many weeks afterwards, mulled it over internally and externally. Tentative plans were made for a visit when the leaves are most gorgeous in the Northeast.

The season progressed with seeing the dentist and going to doctor's appointments, and being referred to a dermatologist after finding out he had skin cancer on his back, face and neck. Being referred sounds simple. Not many dermatologists are interested in taking on a CareOregon/Oregon Health Plan/Medicaid patient. After searching high-and-low for one, I returned to the place that always has helped Tracy: Oregon Health Sciences University. Of course they had a dermatologist available who would be interested in taking care of him. We wound up with the head of the Department of Dermatology, who saw and treated Tracy several times, always with students in tow. Tracy enjoyed visiting with them all. I recall sitting in the treatment room and getting to look out the window at the incredible view from the sixteenth floor of the Waterfront complex. It's the same complex where Tracy met Andy and Amy for therapy, but they are on the ground floor.

Tracy's primary-care physician continued to test and tweak his medications to determine if they could be lessened. One Renal Function Panel which tested various kidney functions indicated several "out of reference" range (too high or too low) components. Because of that, his doctor was not in any hurry to reduce his blood-pressure medication.

Tracy's cholesterol was high. His doctors wanted to reduce it. They switched medication. The results were pretty similar to other medicine changes. His blood pressure was no longer stable. He had difficulty swallowing and he couldn't think or speak clearly. His lack of balance was much worse than usual. He had no motivation to do anything. They gave up and put him back on the previous medication that wasn't as effective, but caused fewer side effects. Tracy still struggles with side effects to medication and, after all this experimentation, he is even more loathe to try "new" treatments.

Social life was picking up. We were viewing more movies and plays and eating more dinners out. Tracy hadn't tossed his cookies for months, except when exercising too hard or getting outside the parameters he had set for himself regarding eye and head movement. In June 2013, we ratcheted up Tracy's physical-exercise program approved by Andy and his doctor. Tracy had morning exercises two to three times a week at the Elsie Stuhr Senior Center. The folks there were great. They taught him how to use their workout machines and mechanical monitors. They worked with him on balance exercises. He became friends with two of the "regulars." Tracy balanced this activity with more walks in Greenway Park, always taking his iPhone so he could take pictures. He showed me all he'd seen on his walks, via photos, when he returned home.

As Tracy settled into this new increasingly difficult physical routine, I noted an interesting change. He was becoming more mentally acute. He was just more "here." I asked him what he was thinking. He said he'd been thinking for months, methodically dissecting information he was given and making sense of what had overtaken him. After processing all that data, he was ready to move ahead and look more outward than inward. He was more interested in what was going on around him than just what was going on inside his head and trying to get his body to come back alive. He still was doing that, too, but he could take on the additional tasks of rejoining the world around him. I asked him if he thought about "going home" to Lincoln City. He looked at me and said, "Always."

Chapter 6:
Nothing Stays the Same...

In mid-June 2013 we received an email from Mary Lou Zeek, an art-gallery owner and friend of Tracy's who had shown and sold his work over several years. She had several of his pieces and was so supportive over the past couple of years. She said she was going in a different direction, "...closing her current gallery and going in the direction of art consulting, artist relations, and concentrating and expanding on outside sales," using her home gallery as a stepping off point. She wanted to keep a few of Tracy's pieces, but needed to make arrangements for us to come by her gallery in downtown Salem to pick up the remaining work.

In another week, I received an email from Robin, dear Robin, Tracy's friend who was storing a garage-full of many of Tracy's treasures.

"Hi Wendy, I want to give you a heads-up about my plans for the fall. I think I have found a roommate (sic) for the fall. She would want to move in during the month of August. And she would need to have the space in the garage to store her things. Or... if she doesn't move in, I am considering renting out my house and getting an apartment for myself, or perhaps even placing the house up for sale. At any rate, I wanted to let you know in plenty of time so that you and Tracy have as much time as possible to find a place for his things. However, things work out I'll let you know for sure as soon as I know!"

Robin hadn't notified Tracy directly because she wasn't sure how he might respond. I'm glad she let me break the news to him, but, Yikes! She had been so kind, and if she needed to make other arrangements it was, after all, her house and her life! I shared the news with Tracy that afternoon. Two hours later, here's what he emailed to Robin under the subject:

Tracy Has a Question!

"Dear Wonderful Robin, Wendy showed me your email, and I am SO grateful that you have shared your space with me and my things. First of all, you are more than welcome to share with me on email. Wendy will share with me anyway, but so that you know, you're welcome to write me. I am improving as time goes by, and my intention is to wander back to the coast for living. Having said this, please let me know if you have any explorations with regard to me, you and your house. You are one of the few, if not only, person I would consider living with. Having said that, I am not yet driving, but have made overtures to that outcome. I would feel secure living with you in your location, but I have to drive yet. Your thoughts on this matter... You possibly have someone in mind, but I would also be interested. I haven't worked out the specifics, but like I said, my intention was to move back to the coast. More area for your input...

"Maybe I should leave it at that for the moment, but I plan on coming down toward the end of July and I will work either before that or at that time to move my mung. Any thoughts you have on the matter would certainly be appreciated. Know that I will be working on storing and moving as you see fit, and in spite of my current condition, I process information at a slower rate, but I think I process! I am including Wendy in this email because she makes sense out of the things I say!

"So I have an iPhone with the current number being a xxx- number! xxx-xxx-xxxx... I may be a bit slow in answering, but just so that you have it!

Sincerely,

Tracy

"Sent from my iPad, but in case you were wondering, I have had a stroke, so take anything I say with a grain of salt! Unless, of course, it is nice."

Three days later, Tracy followed his email to Robin, dear Robin with another to Mary Lou, his friend and art-gallery owner:

"Mary Lou!

I'm very excited for you. You have always been searching for the best solution for those of us who make the distinction of being artists. But being of your particular ilk, you are both the artist and the ceramicist, so you have the distinction of understanding us as artists and what it takes to make the gallery go. You have my total support.

"Given that I am (sic) a unique position with regard to new work, did you have anything in mind that you wanted to keep. I have made strides to get back into painting, and I have, but it will take a little bit more. I am standing at my easel and making friends with my acrylics, and in time I will begin exploring my oil and wax. I'm also not wed to the smaller paintings I have been doing, but there is some familiarity to pursuing these. I have been scanning some even as I text to you, and I will share with you what I have been up to. I am making progress, and in time I will be painting. I will benefit from your input, and on my making a contribution. I hope to have your ear before you retire to your NEW Gallery and your new tasks, but in the meantime, take care and have a great time planning for the future!

Sincerely,

Tracy

"Sent from my iPad, but in case you were wondering, I have had a stroke, so take anything I say with a grain of salt! Unless, of course, it is nice."

In early spring, several neighbors got together and decided to host the first ever Greenway Neighborhood Garden Tour at the end of June. After agreeing it was not to be competitive, we practically killed ourselves going all out: washing the outsides of our houses, planting many new lovelies, edging and mulching, setting up new garden furniture, top-dressing gravel pathways, power-washing driveways. We planned our activities over potluck dinners and get-togethers involving wine and beer. Tracy was in the middle of it all. When we decided we should have posters and garden post cards, he was tasked with making an appointment with owners and visiting each garden to take appropriate photos showcasing their gardens. He put the photos on a disk and delivered it to Linda, our friend and neighbor, who then sent it to Philip, an artist friend of hers in California, to make the cards. Linda got the posters. We put them up and passed them around. On "the day," Tracy was a host in the garden. At the "after party," Tracy was one who told stories about who said what in the gardens during the tour. Tracy's observations were interesting. He knew who needed to sit in the shade and have a drink of water, which he got for them; he knew who was a gardener and who just liked looking at pretty gardens, and he talked with all of them.

About this same time, Tracy was preparing for his presentation on Art and Stroke to the Stroke Survivor Group at Legacy/Meridian Hospital where he attended Daria's speech clinic. Daria and some other staff apparently had discussed the possibility of Tracy speaking on the topic from his perspective. They thought he'd be ideal – if he wanted to do it. I could tell he was pleased to be asked. Tracy pondered the idea for awhile and then said "yes." He researched his art-history books, revisiting earlier work that helped form his artistic temperament. He reviewed hundreds of his paintings, photographs and journals. He narrowed prospective examples of work he wished to share. He began crafting a power-point presentation. He consulted via email with his favorite graduate student who was assisting him in the presentation.

I watched in awe. This was a giant leap ahead from just a few months earlier. I had seen a huge leap forward when Tracy began watching live TV, and this was another great step. The giant leaps were coming faster and becoming more frequent.

On the evening of the presentation, we arrived at the room early and found it transformed. From an around the big table classroom setting, it had changed to having chairs set theater-style, a table of soft drinks and hors d'oeuvres, a big screen behind a podium set at proper height so Tracy could sit comfortably, and excitement permeated the room.

As the time grew near for the start of Tracy's talk, the audience filtered in. Every chair was fllled and there was an overflow crowd standing around the room's edges. It seemed many people had heard about the night's program.

I again was entranced by how people with traumatic head injuries and other physical damage act with each other. I had seen some of these folks before in various settings, and on an off-day – which any and all of them have once in awhile – they can be loud, obnoxious, inattentive, demanding and rude. But not with each other.

Tracy had their attention and earned their respect from the moment he slowly and carefully walked to the podium and began speaking.

He took them on a journey of art, and they gladly went along with him. After awhile, he passed around six twelve-inch by twelve-inch paintings he had completed since his stroke. He invited them to look at them, smell them, and, my favorite, touch them. They had a lively discussion about what the paintings were and what they represented. One man, a truck driver, looked non-plussed when Tracy responded to his question about the meaning of a picture. Tracy said that it was whatever the viewer wanted it to be.

After speaking for more than an hour, Tracy lingered for another hour to talk to people. Many wanted to ask him what he thought about their own experiences. Some said they'd always wanted to do something artistic, and now they felt it would be O.K. if they did. We took Tracy home, a jabbering, exhausted, happy person. Another milestone had been reached.

About this time, Tracy took it upon himself to come up to speed on the status of payments from one of the galleries, where he previously had shown work. The gallery had owed him money for years for paintings already sold. I thought it was great, since it showed tremendous cognitive regeneration on his part. And, if he received money owed to him, that was all to the good. He wrote the following two emails:

July 24, 2013:

"Hello All.

Ron, I assume you are the recipient of this. I continue to get better, but I still have significant issues with my speech and walking, but I am continuing to get better. I trust you are continuing to get better on the basis of your gallery and their sales. What I would appreciate from you is a payment schedule. I hope this has given you enough time to get better financially. I am in the process of trying to paint again, and I could use your sales to help finance my way. As G***** and Wendy came to an agreement, I will follow-up. The total was 4,150.00 and a payment for "Crocodile" was the last payment made (9.30.2011). The total still owed is $3,400.00, based on Gxxxxx's accounting. (Deja Vu, Mood Indigo and South Coyote Butte)

Thank You for time on this matter,"

And on August 19, 2013:

Hello All.

I believe this is for Ron first, but his email was kicked back as undeliverable. I am sending this to G****** in hopes that it will find its way to Ron. Just so that you know, I haven't received a peep from this email. As I said before, I would appreciate a payment schedule. I am hopeful that sales are better, and that repaying me won't be an issue. I think the date of my last message to you was about the 24th of July, and that an answer this week would be nice. We'll see where this goes before my next move.

Sincerely,

"Sent from my iPad, but in case you were wondering, I have had a stroke, so take anything I say with a grain of salt! Unless, of course, it is nice."

Tracy heard nothing in response to these messages, so he sent a third message in late fall, 2013. In that message he cc'd a local TV station, which investigates various local consumer issues. Shortly thereafter, he received a check for the full amount due. There was no message included with the check. It had taken several years, but he was paid.

At the last of July, we took Tracy to stay with friend chef Sharon at "The Sharon Inn" in Lincoln City. We had come to call her home that because she so freely shares her space with visiting friends. I always feel privileged whenever I get to stay with her because I know that famous and talented chefs also have stayed at her home and I can bask in their glow! This time, I returned to Beaverton and left Tracy in Lincoln City for a few days. The visit was a stellar success. He was wined, dined, feted, and his return was celebrated by so many friends. The stillness, the emptiness of our house without Tracy was unnerving. He'd been at our home going on two years, and I knew we'd bring him back in a few days, but I also knew that, eventually, he would return to his beloved Pacific Coast for good.

Chapter 7:
Going Home...

Many phone calls, text messages and long talks among Tracy and his friends while he was staying at Sharon's home resulted in the following email from me to Robin, dear Robin, with the subject heading:

"Tracy and His Move Back to L.C.:"

"*Hi,*

I am so glad you and Tracy are going to be "roomies" at your house. He's so very ready to return to Lincoln City, hook up again with his friends, and get on with his life. It's been a long journey. He is the most sweetly tenacious person I know. Tracy said I should warn you about my Big Sister Syndrome, so here goes! I want to help him make his transition and know when I drive away, I have left him in good shape, ready to go forward.

"Maybe most important for our planning purposes, when would you like to have him move in? I was thinking of the week after Labor Day if that works for you. I wouldn't expect you to do anything about his move other than to let us know where to put his stuff in his room and the kitchen. We will rent a truck to bring everything down and to bring his things from his storage unit. I will put out a "Help!" call to his friends so we can unload.

"Before he moves, there are a lot of things we have to do: bank, medical, pharmacy, transfer his Oregon Health Plan to a new caseworker, etc. They require knowing when he will be moving.

"Because of his limited finances, he will need to apply for food stamps. We'll help him get that squared away. One of the things they insist on is proof that he has a separate, lockable, storage space for his food. Not sure what you would suggest for that, but it could be in the kitchen, or a closet. We just need to identify what/where.

"Do you have a freezer beyond the normal one in the kitchen refrigerator?

If so, could Tracy share in its use? If not, is there a place to put a small chest freezer?

"I'm sure we'll have more questions as we go along, but for now, this gets us started. Thanks!

Wendy

In mid-August 2013 we met Mary Lou, an art consultant and friend of Tracy, for lunch in Salem. We picked up Tracy's art that she was returning, all professionally wrapped and ready to travel.

In later summer, Tracy's days were full: walking, exercising and planning/discussing his upcoming move which had taken center stage in his life. Although wrapped up in the center of his so long dreamed-of move back to the Coast, Tracy paused at one point and asked me, "Are you going to be O.K.?" My heart almost burst with love and pride and appreciation that he'd gotten to the point he could ask such a question. I told him the same thing I had said before as we talked about how he was doing and where he was going. "I will have done my job if you can move back home." What kept him going for all those dreadfully painful, dizzy, hard months was his vision of his beloved Pacific Coast shining in the distance.

Many questions stretching from mundane issues to more important ones needed answers: would his TV fit in his new bedroom? Who would be his doctor? Where was the pharmacy? Was there a bus he could catch near Robin's home? Where could we put a freezer so we could stock it for him? What will his new address be and where is the mail delivered? Is the kitchen big enough for some pots and pans for him? What will he need to cook? How will we stage the move? Where can I get the forms to apply for food stamps? That was a eventual non-starter. Based on his less than $1,000/month disabilty payment, he qualified for $34/month in food stamps. Really? He and his roommate would have to put up with being inspected to prove he had a locked cabinet and separate refrigerator shelf to store all the food that he'd purchase on $34/month. I have to wonder where all these Food Stamp "abusers" are that we hear about on the news. Maybe instead of being abusers, they're just starving.

We needed to accomplish several things before Tracy left our home in Beaverton. Making final doctors' appointments and arranging to transfer his medical care to Lincoln City; transfer of his case from Washington County to Lincoln County so he would remain on the Oregon Health Plan even though he'd change the insurance exchange and care providers; and finding an eye doctor who would give him a new prescription for his contact lenses – CareOregon wasn't interested in paying for either an eye exam or contacts. Tracy had worn contacts for years and had a couple of pairs of older glasses, but to see well, he needed a new prescription because he hadn't had new contact lenses for over a year. The last pair of glasses he purchased was on a long-ago trip to Ljubljana, Slovenia. As I recall, he had a grand time with the lovely young ladies selling and fitting the glasses. To this day, he gets compliments on the style of the glasses. We found an optometrist willing to do a minimal eye exam and provide a prescription for contacts. The transaction was completed in ten days.

The alternative was to find an eye doctor willing to take on a new patient on HealthShareOregon/CareOregon/Oregon Health Plan/Medicaid (never a slam dunk) and make an appointment, request approval from CareOregon for the appointment, be turned down, cancel the appointment, and then appeal. That would take about two years. I found it very difficult to determine what office took care of the medical paperwork, but all those groups or names kept cropping up with regard to health-care requests we made on Tracy's behalf. Interacting in there somewere also was the Oregon Department of Human Services Aging and People with Disabilities and the Employment for People with Disabilities. It was never clear to me who did what. I just know he got the really big things paid for and that was great. All the small things were annoyances, but doable.

About this same time, Tracy's primary-care physician wanted him to undergo a colonoscopy, a procedure new to him. We made the appropriate arrangements and the procedure was done – a good thing since they found some polyps and removed them. He's on a three-year redo plan.

I researched possible new primary-care physicians/healthcare providers in Lincoln City. I found the doctor who subsequently became his physician, but the process wasn't straightforward. His office couldn't make an appointment for Tracy until he was "transferred" in the system. I couldn't start the paperwork until he moved. And, they asked for Tracy's Medicare number. As far as I knew, he didn't have one. He wasn't old enough to qualify for Medicare. He was still on disability. Nonetheless, they needed the number. Changes apparently were in the works. I figured it was either because his birthday happened in the first week of October or he had been on disability long enough that he would be transferred from disability benefits to

Medicare. Thus, Medicare would become his primary insurance, and the State of Oregon's Medicaid program would serve as his secondary plan. But not quite yet.

I called the 800 number for Medicare. The various menu options steered me toward their online service so, I contacted Medicare.gov on line. That didn't work because they couldn't provide a Medicare card for Tracy because he wasn't on Medicare. At the bottom of the website, I found an instruction to go to Social Security if a Medicare number couldn't be provided for the website.

I went to the Social Security office in Beaverton. Maybe you wonder why I got in the car and drove to the Social Security office instead of telephoning them. Well, based on previous experience, it took less time and was less frustrating to drive to the Social Security office, park, go inside, take a number, wait, and ask my question than to wade through the telephone's 800 menu. They referred me back to the Oregon Department of Human Services Aging & People with Disabilities district office.

So I drove a few blocks, and I met Alma. Alma had the answers I needed. After telling her about Tracy's impending move to Lincoln City, she set up the transfer online and told me who to call in Toledo – the town in Lincoln County that housed their district office. She gave me the online address to apply for a Medicare card. I applied and within two weeks, Tracy received his Medicare card. And so I was able to set up an appointment with Tracy's new doctor in Lincoln City.

Something also needed to happen about Tracy's driver's license. It was set to expire on his sixtieth birthday in October and, based on the results of the test done at OHSU, his doctor was not going to clear him to take a driver's test to renew his license. Instead, we applied to extend his handicap parking permit and applied for an Identification Card in lieu of a license. We got the forms signed and trooped out to the Department of Motor Vehicles, where he voluntarily surrendered his license at the same time he requested the parking permit and an ID card. I could tell by the look on his face, this was a sad day. He'd had a driver's license since he was 16 years-old.

Tracy's interest in thanking people for what they had done for him was another example of how fast he was recovering cognitive awareness. He was coming to rely on emails and phone texting to do his major "talking" with people. Tracy said goodbye to Cheryl, his lovely massage therapist. She gave us some ideas of what worked well with him, principally with his head and neck, and we passed that along to Tracy's dear friend, Faith, his massage therapist friend in Lincoln City. He said goodbye to his friends at the fitness center and the friends he'd made in our neighborhood. A week before his move, Tracy sent the following email to his trainers and friends at the Elsie Stuhr Center:

> "Hi,
> *This message is for Diane and Desiree, and Corey and Bob among others.*
> "*I am very grateful for a couple of events. One, I am very happy to have found the Elsie Stuhr Center, but more than that, I am very happy to have met the rest of you. I will continue to pursue my weight training, and with it swimming in the winter months. I am bidding you adieu, but in the process if you want to share any email addresses with me, that would be fine. I may be a bit slower to respond--I was ALWAYS slow to respond, but also, I have a Facebook account, but I can be found at www.tracymacewan.com (not updated in a while!) as well as my email at ****.*
> "*Take wonderful care, and I am sure that Corey will have a cup of coffee on my behalf until later, when I am ready to take a sip for myself! That and Bob adding a few pounds to my lifts!*
> *Tracy*
>
> "*Sent from my iPad, but in case you were wondering, I have had a stroke, so take anything I say with a grain of salt! Unless, of course, it is nice.*"

Tracy and I talked about his Advance Directive. In Oregon, residents have the option of completing a form called an Advance Directive, which allows a person to express his/her wishes for care and life-sustaining treatments if they are unable to speak for themselves. It also allows a person to authorize a "health care representative" to make health-care decisions for them in the event that they are unable to speak for themselves. I wanted him to be aware that he had choices about what medical treatment he could authorize ahead of time should he suffer another traumatic incident. He already had completed a (POLST) form. A POLST is Physician Orders for Life-Sustaining Treatment. This form is actually a medical order, signed by one's doctor, which indicates the types of life-sustaining treatments you do or do not want if you become gravely ill, including cardiopulmonary resuscitation (CPR). This bright pink form is to be placed on your refrigerator so EMTs can find it if they are called to your house. I had never paid attention to these forms before Tracy had his stroke. It was another layer of my education.

We decided that since he was moving back to Lincoln City, Robin, dear Robin, should act as his primary health-care representative, and I would be his secondary representative. These are discussions no one wants to have but we all need to have them. As a result of making sure Tracy had his affairs in order, Bill and I began discussions about what we wanted regarding medical treatment or intervention should we suffer a catastrophic illness. Of course, we got into an argument. I told him I'd do whatever he wanted for himself, just let me know. He didn't like the choices I made for myself. But I made the ones I thought were right for me.

Packing and moving Tracy's things to Lincoln City was a big deal. After his first visit back home, Tracy spent some time on each subsequent trip going through what was in the storage unit and what was at Robin's house. Eventually his couch, pink chair, wetsuit and wheelchair would be moved from Sharon's house where they were on loan or stored. (Sharon's dad used the wheelchair when he visited in the early summer.)

On Tracy's very first visit to his "mung," as he called it, he took many photos. I had thrown nothing away. I felt I didn't have the right to dispose of anything belonging to Tracy. I believed, hoped, prayed that Tracy would again have use for all his things. Oddly, I believed that I maybe wouldn't jinx his recovery if I could keep all his things together. On later visits, he surrounded himself with his "mung," contemplating. Over time, much went to Good Will, the thrift store, or the Artists' Coop. But, it all still had to be sorted, moved or stored somewhere. Tracy thought he could winnow it down so we could empty the storage unit, thus saving one-hundred and ten dollars a month, and somehow get everything into Robin's garage. I had a mental image of a garage with flexible pop-out sides. Robin found friends who had a freezer, so that went into the garage. I brought food for the freezer, and left Tracy pretty well stocked with chicken, home frozen vegetables and homemade jams.

I had a long list to cover before Tracy moved:

Notify Lincoln City Storage that we were vacating his storage unit;

Cancel the insurance on the storage unit;

File for Food Stamps;

Make final appointments with Tracy's Portland-area doctors;

Change his automatic bank deposit for his disability check;

Get a new debit card at the Lincoln City bank branch and notify our branch of changes;

Make motel reservations in Lincoln City for Bill during the move;

Ask for room for Alison and me at the "Sharon Inn" during the move;

Make a Costco run to stock Tracy's larder;

Take coolers;

Ask Paul, our contractor/friend to dismantle shelves, easel and work benches for the move;

And, ask our pet sitter to stop by while we were gone to tend to our two cats.

Just before Tracy's move, I sent the following email to all the parties concerned: "Change of Address:" "Effective 9/7/2013, JTM has a new address: in Lincoln City." I had wondered for so long whether I'd ever again be able to make the statement, "Tracy lives in Lincoln City." It had been two years, two months and 17 days since he left his hometown via Life Flight.

After due consideration, we rented a U-Haul truck and contracted with a Lincoln City moving company, recommended by Sharon, to move all the heavy stuff at the Lincoln City end. After all, Tracy's friends had stepped up in the past, and how many times can you ask people to come help move stuff? Bill got the U-Haul at noon on Thursday, September 5, 2013. We hadn't planned to ask for help, but I'm so grateful to our friends who were supremely helpful on the Beaverton end. Paul, Karla who is a garden designer friend and married to Randy, plus Amador, who sometimes works with Karla – all helped Bill, Tracy, Alison and me make quicker work of emptying our house and filling the U-Haul that afternoon.

Bill left the next morning, driving the truck with Tracy riding shotgun. I followed in a very full car with Alison tucked in around various odd pieces than couldn't go in the truck. We met the movers at Robin's home, and we didn't break any of our Lincoln City friends' backs or give them hernias, as I was afraid we might have done with our friends in Beaverton. Matt, Tracy's friend who used to work at a Lincoln City art gallery where Tracy showed work, came by and lent his energy to moving Tracy in to his new home.

In addition to moving items from our house to Robin's, we also had to clean out the very full storage unit. And, Robin's garage wasn't empty of Tracy's items, either! Tracy and head mover Anthony consulted, eye-balled space (a great way to measure if you can get away with it, and they could and did), rearranged the garage, emptied two truckloads, plus the things from Sharon's house, and they set up Tracy's bed so he could collapse for his regular nap. The weather even cooperated: no rain, and that's not a given on any day at the Coast. We kept a pathway through the garage so Tracy and Robin could serpentine their way through the very crowded space.

On the day after Tracy moved, Robin wrote the following on Facebook: "I'm so excited that my new roommate has finally moved in! My only worry is that the cats seem to love him more than me! And his cozy chair."

Tracy spent the next ten days being feted by friends celebrating his return home and he spent a little time assembling his computer table, putting up paintings in his bedroom and wandering around the garage. He went shopping at BiMart, a local store carrying groceries, clothing, kitchen items and more, with Robin to find various necessary items like peanut butter and happily settled into his new space. We talked each day.

I spent that time being so aware of Tracy's absence. It was "heavily" quiet in our house. Not that he is noisy; he definitely is not. (Stories from his friends indicate differently...) It was the absence of his presence. I kept determinedly busy. I reclaimed his room as a guest room – albeit that it would be "his" guest room whenever he visited, but I cleaned and fluffed and got the walls repaired and painted. I put the living room back together. Soon we would have new laminate floors in the living room and central hallway to replace the very tired wall-to-wall carpet we inherited when we bought the house ten years ago. And the family room was downright spacious with just two recliners in it. I attacked the garden for fall cleanup. Every time I came into the house, it was as if large parts of it were empty. It wasn't that one room or one-third of the space was empty. It was that a part of the whole was gone. But I am so lucky. I lost my brother to the place he loves the most. He's where he wants to be. After all, he moved there fourteen years ago just for a year, to figure out whether he liked it. He just spent two-plus years working his tail off to get back there. This ending is so much more joyous than that for so many others who care intensely for loved ones, only to lose them altogether.

Is Tracy different now? Yes. But it's not all bad. He's gained a peace and joy d'vivre that he strove for previously. It came to him in a most unexpected circumstance, but he has today, in many ways, what others continue to seek.

Tracy and I each celebrated our new-found freedom in the same way. It wasn't planned; it just happened. We both took a trip – to different places. In the past, whenever Tracy or Bill or I traveled alone or together, we would begin the journey singing altogether, "And the Adventure Continues!" And so it did. I went back to Lincoln City ten days after Tracy's move to bring him back to our house on the first leg of his journey to see our cousins in New Hampshire. Over the summer, he had made his travel arrangements, working out details with our cousins. He stayed with them about two weeks. His adventure was not totally boring: the plane was late from Portland, so he missed his connection in New York and had to make catch-up arrangements. He did and he did it well. He said later he purposely didn't let me know until after it was all over because he didn't want to worry me and, he wanted to know he could fix it. I guess if you have to fix something, if you can do it in New York, you can do it anywhere! He relished his visit, catching up with his cousins and getting to know four young additions to the family since he'd last visited and traveling to Prince Edward Island – an annual trek that our cousins make that Tracy's been able to do with them in the past. Being able to retrace steps and rekindle family friendships mattered greatly to him.

Five days after he returned home, I left – on Tracy's birthday – for southern France, also for two weeks. I traveled with his friend, Sharon, and got a chef's tour of France. Tracy house-sat/cat-sat for Sharon while we traveled in France. Sharon and I stayed a few days in Collioure, a lovely small town on the Mediterranean Coast near Spain, and the remainder of the time we were in Provence at a chateau in the middle of a vineyard with a group of her friends – other chefs including Liz and Sally who I had met in Lincoln City the year before. I knew I had died and gone to heaven.

It was such a perfect ending and starting point: the trip to France punctuated the end of active caregiving on my part, and the resumption of my own life. I had the best of all worlds. Tracy could now be a visitor at our home and we could visit him in Lincoln City. The bottom line is, he is still on this Earth. For that, each day, I am so very grateful. Early on after Tracy's stroke, his remaining with us in *this* life was never a given. It took months after he returned to Lincoln City before I didn't wake up at 5 a.m. to get some early quiet time. I no longer needed to. I could loll in bed and watch the sky lighten in the east, listening for frogs, bird songs, and coyotes in their seasonal time. I could listen to the rain outside and not feel required to jump up and do something. And, I could begin to re-establish a softer, closer, less activity-driven relationship with Bill. I knew we had work to do.

Part 3:
Epilogue…

For those of you who check the back of the book first to see how the story turned out...

More than five years later, Tracy still is very much in this world. And I am, too. Each of us has moved into our new "old lives." Mine more nearly resembles what I was doing before. His is more different.

After moving in with Robin, dear Robin, back at his beloved Oregon Coast, Tracy moved again several months later. Robin, dear Robin, found her own true love and Tracy felt that, with Robin's help, he had regained his footing in Lincoln City. It was time for him to move on. Through Sharon, (how is it that she keeps coming through in a pinch?) Tracy found George and Gloria and their downstairs apartment overlooking George's garden and the Pacific Ocean beyond, resting at 101 feet above sea level – one-foot above the tsunami zone. I met George and Gloria as Tracy was considering becoming their tenant – and I'm pretty sure they were doing some considering, too. I gave them my contact information and asked one thing of them: Please make sure you either hear or see Tracy once a day. They said of course they could do that. Tracy looked at them and chimed in, "And I'll do the same for your kids!"

Tracy's life is assuredly different. But "place" remains paramount to him, and he's in the right "place." He continues to make progress, health-wise, contrary to what many in the insurance and bureaucratic worlds prognosticated. He has accomplished something amazing: he's figured out how to accommodate what he cannot accomplish. And he's done it with grace and acceptance. Today, he's as dizzy as he ever was. But he employs techniques he's learned from great therapists to keep himself (mostly) from tipping over, falling downstairs, lurching into bushes, and vomiting. He knows how to pace himself. Daily naps remain a specific reminder of the debilitating fatigue caused by strokes. He struggles with finding and saying the words he wants, but each time I see him, I note improvement in his speech and choice of vocabulary. He mitigates his frustration by emailing and texting more than he used to. Tracy is using his camera to talk for him, and Facebook was made for his current method of communication. Those activities themselves are a win: he's still relearning control of his hands and fingers – above all both hands at the same time. He related what he considered to be a very funny experience. He and his friend Joe were at Sharon's house. Since Sharon is constantly housing guests, anyone who comes by is tasked with checking the dryer to determine whether sheets need to be folded. Tracy found a queen-sized bed sheet that needed folding. As he would get one corner "organized" in one hand, the other hand dropped the opposite corner. When he picked up the opposite corner, the first hand dropped the first corner. He started laughing. This continued until Joe came to the rescue.

Tracy spent more than a year after moving back to Lincoln City circling the realm of abstract painting. He did some painting, primarily acrylic. He finished one piece that he had started before his stroke. It hangs in Volta Gallery on Highway 101 in the Taft part of Lincoln City. He said he felt he was still in "preparation mode." Before his stroke, he used to laugh about being like a dog that circled its bed several times before getting into it. That was the way he launched himself into painting. He was doing the same thing after he returned to Lincoln City but for different reasons. But then, a couple saw his painting at Volta Gallery and they were intrigued. Would he consider a commission for something similar but smaller? He's now completed that commission with the installation of the painting at their home in August, 2015. I believe both he and the couple are happy with the result.

Tracy's treasure is his many friends. They have remained his friends for a reason: They love him. He has friends of long-standing who live all around the country. They are in regular touch. There seems to be a secret network among the friends who live at the Coast: someone is in touch with him just about every day. Some have regular times, like Matt, who has lived in Lincoln City for years with his family and who knew Tracy through an early art-gallery connection, and who now walks with Tracy each Wednesday. Sometimes friends decide it's time for dinner at La Roca, or breakfast at RockFish. Occasionally, Tracy house-sits for friends. Recently, he was house-sitting in a pretty isolated place without good cellphone coverage. His friends just kept popping in. They give him rides on occasion. He's located now where he can walk down the hill to the store and the doctor's office and the pharmacy. He's made friends with the local bus line, and rides to the Community Center two or three times a week for his workouts. He also spends time at his studio at the Cultural Center, the Jennifer Sears Glass Art

Studio, and Volta Gallery.

Not long ago, Tracy was telling a new friend that he really missed driving. On a Sunday, she took him to the local high school parking lot and had him drive her car. He drove around the parking lot and then down the street to the local elementary school. He said it seemed "old hat for me, but I am very appreciative to make my way in the world." Tracy told her that it would be a real boon to have his dependency reduced during the winter – when Lincoln City moves itself around at a much sparser pace. Passing the driver's test and getting – and paying for – insurance are still on the horizon. He moves ahead, cognizant he's not likely to drive cross-country anytime soon, but tootling around Lincoln City on a quest for groceries is a fine activity.

Last year, Tracy wanted to file his own tax returns. He's been keeping records of his income and expenses on Quicken, his check register, and through his credit card. After discussing how it was going, we decided I would bring home his information on a thumb drive and do his taxes. He says a long series of mental steps is still a great challenge for him. The steps slip away so easily mid-way through the journey. In the perverse way of head trauma, he knows, for example, that something is legitimately a business expense, but when asked what exactly it is or does, he could only repeat that it is a business expense. It took several phone calls – exhausting for both of us – to determine things such as what Blurb did for his business and what a FireWire Adapter was.

After writing this story and being told it would be published in 2016, I asked Tracy if he thought he could build a website for the book. He said yes. What a long and incredible journey he's made.

Unpaid lay caregivers are beginning to gain recognition for the critical role they play in patient care and long-term health. It's imperative that capable caregivers are available to patients who are being discharged as soon as hospitals can get rid of them. Oregon recently passed a law to support family caregivers by making sure they are at the table to participate in discharge planning and that they receive post–discharge training for the complex medical tasks they perform for their loved ones, such as wound care, medication management, the operation of assistive devices and injections. Other states, such as New Jersey and Oklahoma, have passed similar legislation.

Finally, because of a lawsuit, Medicare is slowly getting it right, and hopefully other agencies will as well: No standard of improvement is now required for Medicare. That means various forms of therapy are appropriate for the general medical well-being of people like Tracy, irrespective of whether they show measurable "improvement." That's not to say we haven't had Medicare/Medicaid resistance to getting occupational therapy for him. We still have to request "evaluation visits" because we see improvement – which I actually do see. But hey, I'll call it whatever they want me to call it: improvement, applesauce, whatever! We have brought Tracy back to the Portland area in the last year for week-long intense physical and occupational therapy sessions at Oregon Health Sciences University. Above all, Andy, his physical and vestibular therapist, remains a saint in my eyes. Andy tailored the work she had Tracy do personally for him, concentrating on controlling dizziness, focussing strength and coordination and performing multiple simultaneous and divided tasks with a push for speed.

All the exercises are difficult. One exercise, I recall, has Tracy on his hands and knees, simultaneously raising one leg and the opposite arm purposely to trigger dizziness – and then working through it. I'd have trouble doing any one of the things asked of him, such as, hopping back-and-forth over broom sticks, reciting the alphabet backwards and juggling a big fuzzy ball, all at the same time.

Andy explained to Tracy that the reason he was so tired after these sessions – there were four in a week – was that remapping his brain is exhausting, and he recovered and much of the remapping occurred while he slept. Roseann, the occupational therapist, had him juggling (great until he laughed so hard he dropped everything), and picking up small washers and nails or poker chips with both sets of fingers at the same time. She also helped him realign how he stands at his easel, showing him how he was tilting his head back (increasing dizziness and nausea) instead of holding it level in coordination with his trunk and shoulders. I point out these details in hopes that other caregivers will take note: Find professionals because they can help provide direction and evaluate progress.

Tracy also received permission to see his speech therapist, Daria, for an evaluation after more than a year. As she said when he greeted her, she was "blown away" by how good he looked and how much better he was speaking. One assignment she gave him was to recite his own poetry to her on voice mail. He's been reading aloud Maurice Sendak's books and says that reading aloud helps him hear himself so he does a better job of piecing together phrases instead of jerkily throwing words at each other.

For much of the time I watched Tracy "get better," I harbored a continuing resentment. I live in the United States of America. In my opinion, it has a mostly broken health-care delivery system, almost totally based on the premise that who has money – or good insurance – gets access to the best care. I followed the treatment and continuing improvement of former U.S. Representative Gabby Giffords from Arizona after she suffered horrific brain trauma in an assassination attempt. I'm so glad she received the care she did. She absolutely deserved it. I resented that the level and extent of after-care she received was unavailable to my brother. As time went on, however, I realized Tracy had gotten exemplary medical care. He also received superb therapy as he worked on his recovery. I just had to work harder to gain access to it. We were committed to doing much of the treatment and therapy ourselves. As I watched Tracy improve, I concluded that we couldn't have bought better care for him. I became his "access" by finding ways around barriers. I learned many skills.

One of Tracy's long-time friends says he hopes one day he will see Tracy on a TV talk show or in front of a congressional hearing talking about why we need new legislation to provide insurance coverage – sort of a stroke parity – for those who have had a stroke to rehabilitate. Speech limitation remains one of Tracy's biggest challenges. We had little success gaining access to his speech therapist other than through the critical provision of Legacy's free speech clinic. I call Tracy and talk with him specifically because it's harder for both of us. Sometimes we text/email, but I want to hear him talk. He needs to talk, every single day. Listening to him say words like "proximity" and "perfectly" makes me smile.

Tracy continues to amaze me. Whatever the challenge, he takes a breath and recoups. Every morning when he gets up, he has to get up carefully. He has to think about his next moves because when first arising in the morning, he can be more than usually dizzy. But not always, so he has to investigate how he is today. And that's before he leaves his bed in the morning. Sometimes he can't do a particular fine-motor function with his fingers so, the TV remote, the computer mouse and keyboard are the recipient of his frustration. But he says he's still getting better. And I believe him.

As for me, Thanksiving and Christmas continue to be the times of reflection and appreciation for where we are and what we have. They also are times of pure fun when we spend time together seeing plays and musicals, hearing great music, and eating terrific food.

In the summer three years after "The Event," I began to look around to see what volunteer activity I could do because my mind had rested enough. I needed challenges again to earn my keep in the world. After serving as an alternate for six months, the next January I once again joined my local Planning Commission. I've continued to volunteer with my local Park and Recreation District in various capacities, for which I am grateful. My friend, Linda, a delightful combination of artist and gardener, has led me into the world of garden art. Together we have crafted garden totems that tell the stories of our gardens, and we created a piece of art on a big door that acts as a gate in the garden. She believes I'll graduate from being the person who primes to the one who paints, and I love her for it – but I don't believe her! As always, I continue close fellowship with my Bridge Sisters. Many of us have gone through traumatic events in the last few years and it has been unbelievably special that we could care for each other in these times of stress. In every way, I am so appreciative of each day – most happily those without stress.

Did this time take a toll on me? Yes, I think so. Obviously, I grow older, but while my body has more than its share of aches and pains, I believe they might not have been quite as great had I not taken on the physical aspects of caregiving. I offer this observation as a cautionary tale to other caregivers. Carrying or moving heavy equipment, helping to balance a grown man who weighs more than I do, increased cleaning and cooking and generally helping another live his daily life was more than I had been doing. I'm not alone. Many caregivers are of "a certain age" and we all need to be careful not to exhaust or injure ourselves.

So many things still remind me of the time Tracy and I spent together:
The little blue ground cover that flowers every spring under the liquidambar tree next to which Alison sat cradling Tracy waiting for me to come get them after Tracy took them both down on one of their early walks;
The dents and scrapes in the bathroom walls where Tracy learned to manuever the wheel chair in close spaces;
Seeing our local firefighter/EMTs in all their regalia at a neighborhood meeting;
Tracy's red couch that now lives in our living room;
Two round blue plastic throw-up bags that still sit crumpled and ready in

the glove box of my car;
    Tracy's many paintings that hang on our walls;
    Each time I hear a helicopter, thinking of Life Flight.
    The wheel chair, walker, tub chair and toilet seat that now reside in our *attic, hopefully never to be needed again, but kept there to stave off the demons.*
Sometimes after such a reminder, I call Tracy, just because I can.

It's pretty common knowledge that major life traumas test the fabric of relationships and that many unions do not withstand the assault. Bill and I almost lost us. Bill disappeared into his office on his computer, out to meetings and traveling. In the end, Bill produced a published novel. I concentrated on becoming an expert on all things medical and bureaucratic. Neither of us focused on us. Mostly because he didn't want to and I was already used up. We put us on hold. That probably saved us because we couldn't have survived a fight. But there was something else. We both love each other. A lot. Bill said he thought about leaving. But he didn't want to go without me. I couldn't leave.

For those of you who wonder, Bill and I made it. We have too much history to rend the fabric of our life together. It would tear in so many pieces that it would leave each of us in shreds. I wasn't sure Bill would be willing to wait. But he did. Today, we argue over really important things such as whether to leave for a vacation on a Wednesday or a Thursday.

Never again will *life* be the same. But truly, this added layer of time and experience feels more like patina, providing greater depth and shimmer to *life*.

And the Adventure continues.

View other Black Rose Writing titles at www.blackrosewriting.com/books /1nd

use promo code PRINT to receive a 20% discount when purchasing.

BLACK ROSE writing™

CPSIA information can be obtained
at www.ICGtesting.com
Printed in the USA
FSOW03n0830241016
26501FS